Bradford Dementia Group Good Practice Guides

Training and Development for Dementia Care Workers

Anthea Innes

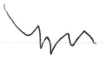

Jessica Kingsley Publishers
London and Philadelphia

The right of Anthea Innes to be identified as author of this work has been asserted by her in accordance with the Copyright, Designs and Patents Act 1988.

First published in the United Kingdom in 2000 by
Jessica Kingsley Publishers Ltd,
116 Pentonville Road, London
N1 9JB, England
and
325 Chestnut Street,
Philadelphia PA 19106, USA.

www.jkp.com

© Copyright 2000 Anthea Innes

Library of Congress Cataloging in Publication Data
A CIP catalog record for this book is available from the Library of Congress

British Library Cataloguing in Publication Data
Anthea Innes
Training and Development for Dementia Care Workers –
(Bradford Dementia Group good practice guide)
1. Dementia – Patients – Care 2. Public health personnel –
Training of
I.Title
616.8'3

ISBN 1 85302 761 8

Printed and Bound in Great Britain by
Athenaeum Press, Gateshead, Tyne and Wear

05212210

Contents

Acknowledgments

There are many people who have helped in some way with my thinking for this guide. In particular, I would like to thank all those at Anchor Trust who have been involved in any way in the Bradford Dementia Group/Anchor training project, which provided the impetus for this guide. Colin Bell, Bob Woods and Ian Jacques made useful comments on drafts of this work. As usual, Tommy and my family provided moral support. The late Tom Kitwood suggested that I write this guide and spent time discussing my early ideas and devising a structure for the guide with me; I would like to dedicate this work to him.

Preface

This guide to good practice is based largely on experience gained through my ongoing work with Anchor Trust, who wish to develop a training capability in dementia care. This has involved working intensively in an Elderly Mentally Infirm (EMI) registered residential home, a nursing home for the 'frail elderly' and a general residential home. Each home has piloted a dementia care training programme introducing the person-centred philosophy of care and applying this to many key areas of care practice, such as care planning and risk assessment. Anchor Homes is soon to begin the 'roll out' of the training package throughout its 97 homes. For this to be effective, both at the micro level in each home and at the macro level of the organization, many key aspects that require consideration for a training programme to have any success are coming to light. The commitment of the manager of the home, 'grass roots' staff and middle management within the organization has proved vital for the adoption of ideas discussed in training to have a positive impact on care practice and the lives of people with dementia. Training and professional development courses, programmes and strategies are not without their difficulties. During the course of my work with Anchor there were many issues to consider during all phases of the programme: when setting it up, when negotiating with staff and when trying to put staff suggestions arising from the training into practice. Factors emerged that appeared to facilitate the development of ideas discussed within training into day-to-day care practice.

This guide draws upon my experiences and is in a sense the result of my personal reflections on the Anchor training work. It also incorporates my experience of delivering short courses with other members of Bradford Dementia Group. Although the guide includes realistic examples developed from my experiences, I have chosen to limit accounts of my own practice. This is because factors unique to me such as my personality, background, gender and class will have influenced my experience of the training process, which others will experience differently. The guide is divided into six chapters, each of which deals with one discrete phase in the training process. Some of these phases often go unacknowledged or unrecognized by those involved in the design or delivery of training. I begin with two chapters suggesting issues that a facilitator should consider prior to the design, delivery or implementation of a training programme. The first suggests broad issues that a facilitator may wish to consider in relation to the home or organization involved in the delivery of the training. The second stresses the importance of getting to know the setting in which the training is expected to have an influence on practice; the main purpose of this is to try to ensure that the training is of direct relevance to the participants in the training programme. The third chapter discusses the design of a training programme, highlighting both theoretical and practical issues. A discussion on the delivery of a training programme follows, which raises practical points for the facilitator to consider. The fifth chapter considers the often thorny issue surrounding the implementation of ideas discussed within training. Practical ways of putting learning into practice are discussed, as are obstacles that may need to be overcome and factors that can help make training relevant and acted upon. This is followed by a discussion on the evaluation of training, both of the programme itself and of whether or not it appears to have had any effect on practice. The final chapter also considers an aspect of the training process that is often overlooked: what happens after the training? How can individuals and staff groups be encouraged and enabled to maintain the momentum gained through training?

While I recognize that each facilitator will find themselves in a unique position, I hope that the many valuable lessons I have learnt in the course of my work with Bradford Dementia Group and Anchor Trust will benefit others who are attempting to develop a training course, programme or strategy for their organization or workplace.

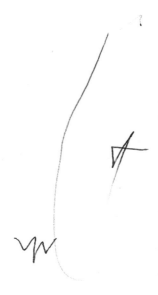

Introduction

The title of this guide alone should suggest that its approach to training and education is not based on what Hyland (1993) has described as 'a quick fix' view of training. A 'quick fix' view of training is that training alone can transform those who receive it. This is a naïve starting point, as the world is a complex place and many factors influence the ways in which people work and live. In the recent past much emphasis has been placed on staff competencies, but little attempt has been made to assess whether the competencies on paper of staff match up to their competence on the job. The National Vocational Qualification model is perhaps the classic example of this concern with paper-based competencies. Effective training involves more than providing staff with necessary skills, attitudes and knowledge, although this may be required. It creates opportunities for participants to draw upon their experiences and helps them develop ways of incorporating new ideas into their current and future practice. The purpose of this guide is thus to outline ways in which training can be used to help staff develop into reflective practitioners.

As well as discussing aspects of the design and delivery of dementia care training programmes, this guide places firm emphasis on the need for the facilitator to think strategically and take into account other factors that may aid or impede the efficacy of an education programme. I argue throughout this text that training is not a magic wand that will solve all problems and resolve all issues within a residential or nursing home. Training, if designed, delivered and evaluated appropriately, may contribute to improving the lives of people with dementia and raise the morale of staff who participate on a programme. However, for training to have a real impact on the way staff work and the care people with dementia receive, the culture of care within a given home often has to change.

Kitwood (1995) argued strongly for a move away from the 'old culture' of care, still evident in homes today in which the focus is on individuals' physical care needs. The new culture of care places the whole person at the centre of the care process. Thus, bodies are not only tended but social and psychological care is provided in an attempt to maintain the personhood, or self, of each person with dementia living in a particular home. Placing the person at the centre of the care process has become known as the person-centred approach to care. This approach is supported by many care practitioners as it offers hope and creates opportunities for the people with dementia for whom they care and also for themselves; this is one of the underlying philosophies of this guide. Different people will have differing opinions on what they consider to be the essential aspects of the person-centred approach to care. However, the aspects of person-centred care I regard as essential are: recognizing and respecting each person's past; recognizing the uniqueness of each person; re-framing 'challenging behaviours' in a positive and creative light; and maintaining communication with each person through the use of verbal and non-verbal communication techniques. If we are to realize Kitwood's vision of a new culture of care, the person-centred approach to dementia care needs to become not just the rhetoric of care providers but the practice of care workers and the lived reality of care provision for all people with dementia.

The other underlying philosophy of this guide is that of student-centred learning. If we hope to achieve care practice that is person-centred then it is not only logical but imperative that staff are treated in a person-centred way. The student-centred approach to education is useful in that it attempts to place the experiences of the learner at the centre of the education programme. This has close parallels with the person-centred approach to dementia care, which places the person with dementia at the centre of care provision. The student-centred approach to training has many implications for the training process. For example, any initial definition of training or education will be influenced by the underlying approach to teaching and learning. Bramley (1991) contrasts the typical British emphasis on individuals' skills, attitudes and knowledge with the American definition of training. The latter places an emphasis on the needs of the organization as a whole, which of course incorporate the training needs of individuals who work within it. Utilizing the strengths of each definition, Bramley suggests that the intention of training should be to improve the performance of individuals and groups within the workplace, which may require changes in the thinking and skills of both. He goes on to argue that training should be a systematic process and that planning is integral to its success. Thus training is part and parcel of developing or creating cultural change within any workplace. Kitwood (1998) discusses attitudes, skills and knowledge training in relation to dementia care. He suggests that training for dementia care work also involves staff reflecting on practice, lowering defensive barriers and developing their practical morality. As such this is an individualistic view of training, typical of the British approach. Training is to promote learning and growth in individual members of staff. It should, in theory, enable them to give more of themselves and be in a position to deliver person-centred care. In addition, however, Kitwood discusses the issue of a 'hidden agenda' within training. This could, perhaps, be the needs of the organization as a whole, and thus reflects the typical American approach to training. While it is vital to recognize the potential for individual growth, development and learning through participation in training, the wider picture must also be addressed. This may indeed be the needs of the organization or the needs of society. It is also important to acknowledge the influence of social, economic and political factors on the residential or nursing home setting, which may create an environment in which training is deemed to be necessary.

Thus I am not only talking about training per se but also about the wider vision of training that any given home or organization adopts. For example, is training part of a programme of opportunities available for staff to take advantage of if they choose, or a compulsory programme that mangers and others identify as necessary to equip their workforce to perform effectively, or a combination of both? If training is presented as an opportunity for staff then individuals may be more likely to be enthusiastic and eager to participate. If training is a compulsory package that staff must work through then it is likely that some people will simply 'go through the motions' and not engage in the process, seeing no personal incentive to do so. Thus, the way in which dementia care training is presented to staff (i.e. as part of a wider training programme or as a specific dementia care training programme) will contribute to the creation of an environment that may or may not be conducive to learning and changing the way in which people work.

If dementia training is part of a specific dementia or wider training strategy it is likely to be a route to a broad and perhaps far-reaching vision of the organization's future. A training programme or course may or may not be part of a training strategy. A training programme can be one or more sessions that set out to improve the attitudes, skills and knowledge of the workforce (which is change at the micro or individual level). Alternatively, it could be a means of achieving change at the macro level instigated by the organization or by a manager within a care setting.

Thus, just as in recent years there has been a move towards person-centred care for people with dementia, there is now a growing recognition that for person-centred care to be achieved the personhood of staff also needs to be recognized. If staff are to participate in training that facilitates the move towards delivering person-centred care it follows that training must be similarly person-centred; this is known in the education world as student-centred learning. If training is viewed as a facilitative process the trainer is in effect a facilitator. The term 'facilitator' is therefore preferred over teacher, trainer or expert, as it suggests that the person who runs and facilitates training is not exerting undue power over the participants. Student participation in the learning process is incompatible with the controlling role traditionally associated with teachers, trainers and experts.

The table below lists four features of the old and new cultures of dementia care and corresponding practices of *trainers* who would be characteristic of an old culture of training and *facilitators* who would be characteristic of a new culture of training. There may of course be discrepancies between training style and the culture of care within a home. A home may operate in a manner characteristic of the old culture of care but the training may be more in line with the facilitative approach appropriate for the new culture of care. Alternatively, the home may be working towards the new culture of care but receiving training delivered in a manner that undermines this approach. It should be remembered that if a home or organization aspires to working within the new culture of dementia care then training should be structured in a manner that supports this.

Table 0.1 Features of the old and new cultures of care and corresponding training practices.

Old culture of care	New culture of care
1. Routines evident	1. Flexible care practices
2. Physical care paramount	2. Social, psychological and physical care of equal importance
3. Care practices geared around staff needs rather than residents' needs	3. Care practices tailored to meet the needs and wishes of each resident
4. People with dementia perceived as inhuman and inferior in some way	4. People with dementia regarded as equal individuals with the same rights as everyone else
Training that would correspond to the old culture of care	**Training that would correspond to the new culture of care**
1. Trainer controls training session and does not give participants a full outline of the purpose of the training	1. Facilitator encourages group participation and clearly outlines the purpose of the training and the desired outcomes
2. Rigid, didactic delivery and teaching style	2. Friendly, open and relaxed delivery and teaching style
3. Content of training places emphasis on controlling residents	3. Content of training places emphasis on understanding residents
4. Trainer provides 'facts' for participants to remember	4. Facilitator provides examples designed to enable participants to draw on their own experiences.

This guide outlines six phases of the training process that I believe are required if training is envisaged as a means of achieving the new culture of care. Six phases may appear daunting and perhaps an extra burden on top of the already demanding work involved in care service provision for people with dementia. However, each phase can, be worked through relatively painlessly if forward planning and strategic thinking are employed. In my experience the benefits gained from each phase of the process have helped in the subsequent phases, which of course increases the probability of a successful outcome for all those involved.

Chapter 1

Getting Started

Prior to the design or implementation of a training programme it is important for the facilitator to familiarize themselves with the organization financing the training and then to begin to get to know the individual care setting(s) where participants work. This is what I have named the 'getting started' phase of the training process. The importance of this initial phase cannot be underestimated: the foundations of good working relationships can be established; the purpose of delivering training to a particular group of staff can be clarified and any 'hidden agendas' uncovered; and the style and methods of teaching/ delivery can be discussed. As this 'setting up' phase progresses, the facilitator will also begin to get a feel for the politics of the organization and the culture of the care homes that the training participants work in. The politics and culture of the organization and home may be blatant or subtle; the possible effects of training on the delivery process, the willingness of staff to participate, and their ability to use and develop ideas within their daily care practice may require careful consideration. This phase is often not acknowledged by those involved in the training programme, but it has a great influence over all the subsequent phases.

ESTABLISHING GOOD COMMUNICATION BETWEEN ALL THOSE WHO WILL BE INVOLVED

An open dialogue between those identified as the key players in the design, delivery, evaluation and implementation of ideas is imperative early on in the development of the training programme or strategy. This will lay the foundations for good communication channels and clear identification of the roles and responsibilities of all those involved. The identities of the key players in the process of the training will vary and may be difficult to ascertain at an early stage. However, it should be possible to identify the individuals who will be responsible for launching the training within an individual care home, a group of homes or an organization as a whole. Key players will certainly include the training programme facilitator, the purchaser, managers involved in the day-to-day running of care settings, and, if the training is part of an organizational, strategy managers at the organization level. The roles of each of the key players may vary. It is useful to consider not only the role of each person involved but how the differentiation of roles will affect the training process. It is also advantageous to examine previous successful and unsuccessful implementation strategies within a home or organization. For example, is a top-down approach necessary for action to be taken? When is a bottom-up approach necessary? For the successful implementation of training it is likely that a combination of both approaches will be necessary. Support is needed from 'grass roots' staff if ideas generated through training are to be developed into care practice. If support is required from management, who may be used to operating within a top-down framework, then this approach may also be needed.

ROLES

The facilitator of the training is obviously a key player in the delivery of the training. If the training is to be relevant to a setting and if the facilitator can draw strongly on their experiences of dementia care then they may also design the training materials. If the facilitator is not involved in the design of the materials then they should, at the very least, be fully informed about the logic behind the structure of the programme and the design of the materials. It may be that the facilitator will use existing materials but design the structure of the training sessions. Those who participate in the training will evaluate the training from their own perspectives; in addition, the facilitator can also evaluate the training according to their perceptions, aims and expectations of the process. Senior managers within the care setting or organization may also be involved in the evaluation of the training. Evaluating the successful development and incorporation into care practice of ideas discussed within training may be the responsibility of the facilitator, home managers, managers within the organization or individuals within the organization who have a responsibility to assess, for example, quality standards within homes. It can therefore be seen that individuals, for example the facilitator of the training and the manager of a home, may have central but differing roles within the overall training strategy (see Table 1.1). The facilitator has a responsibility to deliver and evaluate the training from their perspective and will be involved to some degree in the design of the training itself, whether of the materials or the structure of the training. The manager of a home may be required to plan for staff attending training, attend themselves, evaluate the training from their own perspective and assess the success with which ideas are developed for use in care practice. Therefore, clarification of the responsibilities and role of each key player may be difficult and involve negotiation, but is essential in order to avoid or minimize later ambiguities.

Table 1.1 Possible roles in the training process

Possible roles of the facilitator	Possible roles of the manager of home
Evaluates care setting	Identifies need for training
Designs training	Responsible for implementing training
Delivers training	Evaluates training from own perspective
Evaluates training	Identifies subsequent training needs

It may be that the facilitator of the training is also the manager of the care setting. If this is the case it is possible that the manager will need additional support and that a steering or support group will be necessary. A support or steering group for the training is useful regardless of the identity of the facilitator, as it creates a source of support for all key players in the process.

At the early stages it is very easy to miss out one or two people who may be key players in helping to develop and implement the training strategy. It may be that individuals who are crucial to the success of the training emerge during the delivery or evaluation phases of the training strategy; they can then be brought into later discussions. It is likely that regular meetings will be necessary to ensure that questions can be asked, unforeseen problems discussed, ideas debated and action plans developed. If the role or responsibility of an individual changes or develops over time everyone needs to be notified.

Those involved in the setting up of the training programme will have different skills, knowledge and strengths. A great opportunity is thus created for individuals to pool resources and build effective working relationships. In order to maximize the strategy or programmes success it is vital that members share their knowledge and expertise. However, if time is not invested in developing effective working relationships individuals may be wary and unwilling to do this. This may then hinder the development or implementation of the training at a later date. When there is goodwill towards the training from all those involved it is likely that communication will be easier to establish and maintain. Goodwill should not, however, be taken for granted, as this in itself could lead to the loss of support for the training.

PURPOSE OF TRAINING

What are we trying to achieve by training people? What is the purpose of a training initiative? It may be to give staff basic knowledge, for example of the different forms of neurological impairment that the term 'dementia' covers, or it may be to give staff particular skills training, for example in the use of hoists. However, training may be part of a wider aim of the organization and/or the local care setting to help develop a certain kind of staff group and way of working. Benner's book *From Novice to Expert* (1984) has sparked considerable debate in the nursing world as to what we should be aiming to achieve through learning and development. Is training a way to develop staff into 'experts'? This has been hotly contested within the nursing profession, particularly, as there is no agreed definition of what constitutes an expert (Derbyshire 1994; English 1993; Jasper 1994). The term 'expert' could be taken to imply that the person with this title does not require any further training or professional development opportunities, and can go no further. Alternatively, it could be perceived as meaning that the person has particular skills and knowledge in one area but requires further support and development opportunities to progress in others. However, the use of the word 'expert' can be detrimental to those who are not generally considered to be experts. Certain groups of experts can define themselves in opposition to the non-expert through their participation in training programmes. For example, nurses could claim to be experts because they have received training that care assistants have not. Training can then be seen as a route to status, and can be used to define work roles and tasks in a way that may or may not be fair to all those working in a setting and may have a positive or negative impact on the recipients of care provision. If training is perceived as a means of helping those who participate to develop their skills and abilities rather than as a way of creating this kind of expertise then Benner's notion of developing from novice to expert is unhelpful.

An alternative view can be found in Schon's work on reflective practitioners (1983; 1987). Reflective practitioners may have 'expertise' in a particular area at a particular moment in time, but the ultimate aim is to encourage and enable practitioners to reflect on their experience through training and on their training through experience. Thus, an alternative framework within which to consider the purpose of training and education can be found in Schon's work, in which the purpose of education is considered to be the creation of reflective practitioners rather than technical experts. If reflective practitioners were valued above experts, this would suggest that expert groups would be less able to determine their own and non- experts' roles and tasks on the basis of their training. Rather, the ability to reflect on the training, and its relationship to practice, and vice versa, would be considered a valuable outcome of training. Schon further suggests that ordinary bureaucracies may resist a practitioner's attempt to move from a model of technical expertise to one of reflective practice, and that organizations suited to reflective practice may differ in many respects from bureaucratic organizations (1983, pp.328–9). This is an important point for the facilitator and others involved in training within the home or organization to consider. Will the desired outcomes of the training be supported or thwarted by the current structure and culture of the workplace? In order to judge the ultimate success of the training, it is useful if not vital for those who are developing the training programme to consider, even if only briefly, what they are hoping to achieve by giving staff training. If the development of technical experts is the desired outcome, would it be wise to adopt a training programme which aims to develop reflective practitioners who question and reflect on their practice and then go on to question and perhaps criticize their work culture? Similarly, an organization that wishes to develop staff who are reflective and creative would have to consider the appropriateness of adopting a didactic training style which imparts the technical knowledge staff require to become technical experts. This guide argues that a valuable outcome of training is the emergence of a process of personal development for training participants.

IS THERE A 'HIDDEN AGENDA' TO THE PROCESS?

The original purpose of the training programme may have been part of an organizational strategy to equip the workforce with the skills necessary to meet organizational objectives. For example, the organization's objective may be to promote itself as a provider of good-quality dementia care. If the manager has identified the need for training they may have other concerns that they hope the training will address, such as a need for more teamwork. The facilitator may, when evaluating the setting (discussed in chapter 2), have identified a culture in which it will be virtually impossible for the message of the training to be carried into the care setting without changing completely the way people work. Thus, the actual title of the training programme and its explicit agenda may differ from its implicit agenda. This is known as the 'hidden curriculum' in educational work. Illich (1971) sees schooling as a subversive activity in that it is a way to thus control individuals and shape society. A simple way to illustrate the role of education in meeting the wider needs of society is the extension of formal education. The increase in the number of years children spent in education coincided with technological innovations that lead to fewer employment opportunities; the result of this increase was that unemployment appeared to be less of an issue. Therefore, education in any shape or form is likely to have more than one agenda. The first, that of giving staff 'dementia care training', is made explicit; other implicit agendas may be team building, or developing a marketing tool to encourage clients to choose a particular home or organization. Illich's opinion about education may be viewed as extreme, but it is possible to perceive training as a way of trying to shape individuals in some way. For me the aim of training is to help care staff develop into reflective practitioners; this is essentially an empowering process but could be viewed as dangerous, for example by organizations that wish to have a subservient workforce who do not question and reflect upon their practice.

The training may also be an opportunity for participants to pursue their own 'hidden agendas'. The explicit reason for a manager's participation may be to develop their practice; the hidden reason may be to score 'brownie points' within the organization by presenting themselves as keen to develop and move forward, or to market themselves locally to attract more clients. There may be many personal agendas being played out; Burnard (1989, p.114) suggests that stifled conflict, competition and rivalries can come to the surface within the training session. For example, if there are two or more assistant managers within a care setting they may not work in harmony, using complementary skills and qualities, but instead always be trying to 'get one up' on the other in their day-to-day practice. The same way of working can emerge within a training session, with the persons concerned striving to get others to agree with their view and in the process putting down the person they see as a rival. It may be that there is a divide in the staff group, with two or more factions in existence; these divisions can also emerge within the training session, perhaps preventing members from different groups from working together.

Burnard (1989, p.115) suggests two ways in which the facilitator can deal with hidden agendas:

1. To allow the hidden agenda to play itself out between the members of the group.

2. To invite the group to explore the hidden agenda that is emerging.

If interpersonal issues emerge within the training session it is often possible to intervene in either or a combination of the ways outlined above. For example:

Case Study

The participants are working in small groups, discussing the rights and responsibilities of various groups of people connected with the care setting. One group, comprising members of the senior team and other staff, raises concerns about the way in which the senior team operates in the workplace. The facilitator chooses to leave the members of this group to work through the issue on their own. When the small groups provide feedback to all participants the issue is raised again. The facilitator creates space for an open discussion of the issues.

However, there are hidden agendas that may not be possible for the facilitator to either identify or address. Hidden agendas emerging within the training session can be addressed, although they may remain unresolved. It may be more difficult to uncover and address a 'hidden agenda' on the part of the sponsors concerning the purpose of the training. Dementia care is, at the present time, a developing area. Training may be perceived by the sponsors as a 'quick fix' to plug gaps in the skills of the workforce. If training is used to address such gaps the organization can use training as a means of promoting itself. The organization may be unwilling to explore the impact of the training on staff or the benefits provided to the people with dementia who the newly-trained staff care for. Care provision is a competitive market that is constantly evolving and developing, and as such if it is not necessary now to evaluate and illustrate the impact of training on the workforce and client group, it will be in the future. If homes and organizations are willing to assess the impact of training on staff and people with dementia then it would be appropriate for this aspect of training to be part of the explicit agenda of training programmes.

AGREEMENT AND CLARIFICATION OF THE AIMS AND OBJECTIVES OF THE TRAINING PROGRAMME

Following a discussion of the broad purpose of a training programme and, if possible to become aware of any 'hidden agendas', the specific aims and objectives of training require clarification. The need for a training programme may have been identified in a number of ways, two of which are outlined below:

1. One or more senior managers within an organization may identify the need for a training *strategy*. If this is the case, it is vital that the aims and objectives of the strategy are agreed upon by the steering or support group of key players, in the first instance to ensure that a picture can be sketched for others who are to be involved in the training strategy. The emphasis on the training strategy being a 'sketch' is important at the early stages, as it enables a process of discussion to ensue with those who will receive the training programme and be responsible for the implementation of the ideas it generates. Discussion of the aims and objectives of the programme before its design creates the opportunity to raise

awareness of ambiguities and difficulties that may be encountered. If a training strategy has been identified it is likely, but by no means certain, that there are people within the organization who recognize that training is not a 'quick fix' (Hyland 1993). For the training programme to be effective it may be necessary to have systems in place to respond to issues that arise as a result of the training. A specific training programme that has links with an overall organizational training strategy with the objective of training to meet organizational needs does not automatically lead to support at the local level. It is imperative that those who will receive the training and be responsible for future care provision at the local level are fully briefed and included in discussions at an early stage.

2. Alternatively, at the local level – the care setting itself – the manager or any of the staff working there may have identified a need for staff training in the areas of skills, attitude or knowledge. This works on a narrower definition of training than that discussed above, which incorporates the needs of the organization as a whole. This has its benefits: as training is geared to the individual and local political levels it may be easier to develop a programme that has direct relevance to the particular care setting and meets the developmental needs of those working there. However, it may be difficult to get support from the organization as a whole to implement the ideas developed during the training programme.

Whatever the scenario, be it one or a combination of the two outlined above, it is necessary for the aims and objectives of the training programme to be clarified. Agreement is required between those who have identified the need for a training programme, the purchaser (who may or may not have identified the need) if a facilitator is being 'bought in', and the person(s) commissioned to develop the training programme. The facilitator of the training programme will require information about its aims and objectives even if they are not involved in developing learning materials or the structure of the training programme.

TEACHING STYLES

It is often useful to discuss at the outset with those identified as being crucial to the success of the training programme or strategy the teaching style upon which the training will be based. Teaching styles may be influenced by what is considered to be a desirable outcome, for example, whether the programme aims to produce experts or reflective practitioners. It is widely recognized that different people learn in different ways. Honey and Mumford (1982) developed a questionnaire on learning styles when trying to identify the ways in which individuals (who were, in their development work, managers) learn. Individuals can use the questionnaire to identify for themselves their preferred learning style. Honey and Mumford (1982) suggest that there are primarily four types of learner.

1. The *reflector*, who likes time to think issues through

2. The *activist*, who prefers to learn by 'doing'

3. The *pragmatist*, who tends to be quite practical

4. The *theorist*, who tends to think logically and in sequential steps.

However, it should be remembered that individuals' learning styles will often incorporate elements of all four basic approaches to learning. It is therefore useful for a facilitator to consider ways to incorporate exercises and materials that correspond to all of the above approaches to learning so as to meet the preferences of every participant. In addition, a facilitator should bear in mind that adult learners require particular consideration. There is a vast literature exploring the needs of adult learners and the wealth of experience they bring to the training situation (Knowles 1970; Cross 1981; and Rogers 1986; provide interesting insights). This again suggests a need for the facilitator to consider the many teaching methods and styles available and to decide which will be appropriate. Discussion of these points between all those involved in the training programme may help to prevent conflicts of opinion at a later stage, when misunderstandings concerning the delivery of the training programme may occur. (There is a fuller discussion of these issues in chapter 3.)

THE POLITICS OF THE ORGANIZATION

Training, of course, does not take place in a vacuum. It can be extremely easy to overlook organizational politics that may be instrumental in the success or failure of a training initiative. A facilitator who is an 'insider' may have knowledge of the politics of the organization that a commissioned 'outsider' would not. There are, however, general points that a facilitator may find useful to ponder when considering the politics of an organization. For example, what were the circumstances surrounding the decision to develop a training strategy? Are there certain people who will help to implement the training programme? Who are the people who may object to the training and what obstacles can they create?

Politics operate at different levels within any organization, be it a private company owning between one and five homes, a social services department with many homes in its locality, or large voluntary or private company with many homes dispersed across a wide geographical area. To make a crude distinction, the organization as a whole will have objectives, policies and procedures that individual homes should, in theory, adhere to; at the same time the politics and culture of each individual setting will be unique in some respects. Similarly, while MPs and local government councilors from the same political party work towards the same broad objectives, there are often differences in how councilors will operationalize these at the local level. The facilitator of a training programme has to be aware of different motivations not only for initiating a training programme but for participating in training (either voluntarily or under duress), and training may be perceived as a means of achieving many underlying agendas (outlined above). This is similar to Ovretveit's suggestion that an evaluator needs to understand the interests of different individuals and groups involved in an evaluation (1997, p.188). If a facilitator explores the different interests of those involved in the training process this should, in theory, enable them to make an informed decision as to:

1. whether it is possible to meet the explicit and implicit interests of those involved in the training

2. whether it is desirable to place themselves in such a position.

THE CULTURE OF THE ORGANIZATION

Recent organizational literature places great emphasis on understanding the culture of organizations as an integral part of understanding organizations as a whole (Dawson 1996, p.146). Culture refers to the norms, beliefs and values of the organization. Just as the politics of the organization can differ at the local and global level, so can the culture of the organization (discussed in depth in Handy 1993, chapter 7). The training strategy envisaged at the overall organizational level may not fit the culture of the care setting. Research into the culture of care settings provides insights into care work practices and ways of working. Hockey's work (1990), for example, provides fascinating insights into the impact the physical layout of a nursing home had on the care of dying residents. Residents whose death was considered to be imminent would be moved closer to the matron's office and further away from other residents. The feelings invoked in staff by the care of dying residents or residents thought to be dying, and the space residents who died occupied all affected care practice. The power that care assistants exert over residents' lives and the potential for abuse of that power is discussed by Lee-Treweek (1997). This study exemplifies the paradox inherent in care work: care assistants are relatively powerless within society but are able to control and exert power within the care setting.

These studies highlight issues that may be unique to the individual settings but may also be generalized to other care settings, given that the culture of care work in general is influenced by wider social and economic factors. For example, the reasons care staff give for choosing care work – convenient location, extra cash, hours compatible with domestic commitments (Willcocks, Peace and Kellaher 1987) – will influence who will choose to be employed as a care worker. Wider social factors, such as what is conventionally viewed as women's work and gendered notions of what care involves, play a part in creating the culture of a care setting. In addition, the preferred management style of a home or organization has an important influence on the culture and politics of a setting.

Phase 1 of the training process may help the facilitator to prepare for subsequent phases for the following reasons:

- Communication channels and support systems for key players in the training process are established

- An understanding of the politics and culture of the organization and home emerges

- There is clarification of and agreement on the purpose of training; this includes discussion of 'hidden agendas' and attempts to establish what will be regarded as a successful outcome.

Chapter 2

Getting to Know the Setting

Before implementing a training programme in a workplace, it is of huge benefit to the facilitator to get to know the setting, the residents and the staff group, even if only a cursory impression can be formed at an early stage. This 'getting to know the setting' phase of the process, in my experience, flows naturally from the previous phase. It is not enough to begin to 'get to grips' with the organization as a whole. The care setting itself may be very different from descriptions in documents produced by the organization describing the service provided. Getting to know the setting is important as it enables the facilitator to gain a number of insights into the way in which staff work; these insights can then be used to make the training as relevant to those who will participate as possible. In addition, the facilitator will have the opportunity to assess, in a small way, the training needs of the facility. There are a number of ways to do this. If time allows, it is advisable to conduct a thorough assessment of the setting. When assessing the setting the facilitator should ideally look at both the *processes* of care evident within the home and the *structures* within which care is given and received. Traditionally, structural aspects of care have been examined using checklist-type audit tools; the processes of care have been explored through the observation of interactions between and among staff and people with dementia. Becoming familiar with both processes and structures of care not only provides the facilitator with real information that can be used to back up realistic examples within training sessions, but also provides a kind of 'baseline' measure against which to evaluate the efficacy of the training at a later date (see chapter 6). This chapter explores four ways to get to know the setting:

- Conversation

- Observation

- Audit tools

- Working within the setting.

CONVERSATION

Conversations can take many forms, from an informal chat to a semi-structured or highly-structured interview. Structured interviews often use the format of a questionnaire. The interviewer asks each person a number of pre-set questions and makes notes or ticks boxes throughout the interview. Semi-structured or unfocused interviews are more flexible, with the interviewer tending to use an interview schedule containing a list of topics they wish to explore. The list of topics may be a written or mental list that the interviewer uses to remind themselves of the areas they are interested in exploring. For example:

Warm up question

1.   How long have you worked here?

Main questions

2.   What do you like about your work?

3.   Is there anything you dislike about your work?

4.   What does your work involve? (e.g. What do you do on a typical day?)

5.   Why did you get into care work?

Depending on the context, the facilitator may choose to take notes as they talk or perhaps to record the conversation. It is possible that most conversations will occur during staff tea breaks or when staff are engaged in tasks such as folding the laundry. It would be inappropriate and perhaps impossible to record these conversations as they occur, but the facilitator can write down any key points that emerge soon afterwards.

There are many people who live and work in care settings, and thus the facilitator has access to many potential sources of information. It is important that the facilitator includes both staff and people with dementia in the interviewing process. Staff and resident groups will have different reasons for working or living in the same setting, as will individuals within the staff and resident groups. Goffman's (1961) classic exploration of institutions is a useful theoretical base upon which to explore the care setting. Goffman highlights the differing realities of life in institutions for staff and 'inmates'. An obvious difference is that the setting is the workplace of staff but the home of 'inmates'. In addition, the rights and responsibilities staff may expect for and of themselves may be detrimental to the rights of residents. There is potentially much scope for conflict within any institution in which one group has power over another. It is often easy to assume that the 'inmates' or residents may be the powerless group, but residents can use resistance strategies and thus exert some power and control over staff and their own lives. It has traditionally been assumed that people with dementia cannot be consulted verbally about their views on the care they receive. Thus, interviews are often held with staff but not with people with dementia. However, there have been advances in recent thinking about communicating with people with dementia. Goldsmith (1996), for example, has suggested numerous ways in which we can try to communicate with and hear the voice of people with dementia. Structured interviews may not be appropriate, but informal interviews taking the form of conversation may provide valuable information. The interviewer not only listens to the words of the person with dementia but notes their body language and tries to pick up on the general meaning of their words. This is a much more productive way of trying to hear the views of people with dementia, as noting their exact words could produce sentences that appear meaningless and bizarre. John Killick (1997) has used poetry to communicate the words of people with dementia to a wider audience. If the same words were written in the form of interview transcripts they could appear meaningless; however, his skilful and sensitive use of these words in the form of poems gives the reader a real feel for what the person with dementia is trying to communicate.

If possible, the facilitator should also talk to relatives of residents. Relatives' perspectives on the home will inevitably be partial given their limited involvement in the care setting. They will not be there 24 hours a day, and even if they were it is likely that they would only have contact with their relatives and any members of staff involved in their relative's direct care. They can, however, give their opinion on the care they think their relative receives, the building, and how they think their relative feels about the home. For example:

Case Study

Monica visits her mother every Sunday afternoon in the communal lounge, where hymns are sung with gusto by residents and staff. She often stays for tea before she drives home.

'The staff here are great, they get everyone to join in and there are always cakes at tea time, which my mum likes. My mum always seems happy when I visit.'

Monica's contact with the home is limited to one afternoon a week. From this visit she has formed a very positive view of the home based on the singing of hymns and the provision of cakes.

Case Study

Kevin drops in at the home to see his grandmother each day, either on his way to or from work, depending on his shift.

'*It's OK here, but like anywhere, I suppose, it has good and bad points. Gran gets down quite a lot and on the morning shift staff don't seem to notice, as they are in and out of other residents' rooms. They don't seem to see how she feels.*'

Kevin has greater contact with the home and recognizes that it is 'good' in some respects but not so 'good' in others. In addition, his view is influenced by seeing his grandmother 'down' and this going apparently unnoticed by staff.

The interpretivist school of thought (Hammersley and Atkinson 1983 give a succinct account) highlights the different meanings and interpretations that individuals place on events and situations. This is of relevance to a facilitator who is trying to get to know the care setting. The management team within a care setting may have a different view of the workplace from care assistants, who again may have different views from domestic staff. Residents will have yet another view of the care setting, as they live rather than work there. Therefore it is extremely important to talk to as many people as possible in whatever way possible so as to ensure that the many versions of the reality of life in the home can emerge. For example:

'This is a lovely home, the best place I've ever worked. It's a lovely building and we work as a team.'   (*Manager*)

'I enjoy my work but I don't agree with the way that people are treated differently. We should all be treated as equals and so should the residents'   (*Care assistant*)

'I don't know where this place is. They say I live here but it's not my mother's.'   (*Resident with dementia*)

'The building is always clean and the food looks good. They [residents] don't get out much though.'

(*Volunteer visitor*)

Resource constraints may dictate the number of people the facilitator will have the opportunity to talk with, the length of time that can be allocated to such conversations and possibly the formats conversations will take. It is, however, important that the management team of the setting in which the training programme will take place are involved. Of equal importance is the need to make contact with 'grass roots' staff. This may help to prevent the potential problem of alienating any staff group. For example, the manager of a care setting may perceive the training to be against their interests, or care staff may see the facilitator as part of management and a potential 'spy'. The facilitator has a responsibility to be open and honest about their role within the setting and to address any concerns or queries staff may have. Initial conversations with staff can form lasting impressions, so it is important for the facilitator not to erect false barriers between themselves and those who will participate in the training programme. There are similarities with the person-centred approach, which advocates the need to break down false barriers between people with dementia and care staff. If staff are to break down these barriers between themselves and people with dementia it is also appropriate to break down barriers between staff and trainers. Staff are by no means the experts when it comes to the views of people with dementia on the care they receive; similarly, facilitators are not the experts on the practices and experiences of care staff. Everyone involved in the care or training experience has strengths and knowledge to share as well as weaknesses and 'hang-ups' that form part of the 'baggage' they carry around with them. The facilitator can explore this with staff and in the process uncover their views on their own training and development needs.

OBSERVATIONS

There are many ways in which the facilitator can observe the setting. Unstructured observation can be used. This entails observing the 'whole' setting as far as is possible and taking mental notes to be written up as soon as possible after leaving the setting, or if possible taking notes as you go, so long as this can be achieved in an unthreatening manner. Unstructured observations can provide the facilitator with general impressions of the setting and can be useful in developing a structured observation checklist. Often, however, they can be very time-consuming, as it may take some time to identify the key points that may inform the training programme. Although unstructured observations can inform various phases of the training process it is a good idea to make use of one or more of the many structured observation methods that have evolved over the last 10–20 years. These methods are based on years of work and development, and provide a framework within which to observe the care setting and get at the real dynamics or processes of care.

Brooker (1995) provides an overview of such observation methods, including MacDonald, Craig and Warner's (1985) Short Observation Method (SOM), which looks at activity and behaviour levels, Bowie and Mountain's (1993) Patient Behaviour Observation Instrument (PBOI), which explores behaviours that patients engage in, and Dean, Proudfoot and Lindesay's (1993) Quality of Interactions Schedule (QUIS), which attempts to assess the quality of staff–resident interactions. These are useful starting points for anyone new to observation methods. The SOM and the PBOI both look at the *quantity* of behaviours rather than the quality of the care process. The QUIS attempts to look at the *quality* of interactions, but over short time periods, and as such has the potential to miss details that could have a marked effect on residents' quality of care and quality of life. The method I prefer and which many people are now using to gain insights into the care setting is known as Dementia Care Mapping (DCM) (Bradford Dementia Group 1997, Kitwood and Bredin 1992b). This method has undergone considerable development since it was first taught to people in 1992. The current (seventh) edition of the manual incorporates the recommendations of many experienced mappers. DCM aims to evaluate the setting as far as is possible from the point of view of the persons with dementia who are observed. It looks at the behaviours of people with dementia and attempts to evaluate the well-being or otherwise of each individual person who is observed. Thus the *quality* and *quantity* of behaviours are recorded. DCM has been used by others to assess training needs and can be used as a training tool in itself (Brooker *et al.* 1998; Wilkinson 1993), as DCM involves not only observing and recording information but sharing this with staff to raise awareness of care practices and their effects on people in their care. Ultimately, if staff choose to do so, DCM can also be used to formulate an action plan. It is the observation method I favoured initially when getting to know care settings in which a new training programme was to be introduced, and has proved useful in a number of respects. The usual benefits of DCM – getting a detailed snapshot of the lives of the persons observed which can be used to inform examples used during training – were complemented by insights into the culture of care and work within each of the care settings. It was possible to gain insights into the typical work patterns of staff. For example, I gained knowledge of the tasks they completed in the course of their work, the time of day they appeared to have time to spend with residents, the residents they appeared to have difficulty communicating with and the residents they appeared to enjoy working with. Insights such as these can be very useful when delivering the training as they provide the facilitator with an understanding of the difficulties staff face in their day-to-day work. Obstacles staff may have to overcome if they wish to change the way they work and incorporate ideas discussed within training sessions can also be brought out.

Whatever formal observation method is chosen, it is important to brief staff on the purpose of the observations and to provide information about the people who will be observed, and where, and at what times observations will take place. Those who use DCM do this as a matter of course. Other observation methods do not specify that staff should receive any briefing on the nature of the observations. For research purposes, observers may not wish to give too much away, as they may then contribute to what is known as the Hawthorne Effect. This occurs when those being observed say what they think the observer wants to hear or may behave in uncharacteristic ways. Whether to tell people about observations is therefore a methodological, personal and ethical issue; however, it is impossible to ascertain whether the presence of the observer alone has an effect on the setting. It could be argued that providing participants with information may decrease the likelihood of the Hawthorne Effect if the observer is honestly trying to get a picture of the way in which people in the setting live and work.

The forms observations take are likely to be influenced by time and resource constraints. Indeed, an outsider commissioned to undertake training with a staff group from a variety of care settings in one organization may be unable to visit all the settings. In addition, what is observed and the interpretations placed on observations will be influenced by the observer's contact with and knowledge of the setting and the organization. The view an insider has of the care setting may be quite different to that of the outsider who, at least initially, is likely to view the setting as strange and question events an insider may take for granted. An insider viewpoint does have advantages, as the insider may have greater access to the whole of the care setting and may be aware of the history and context surrounding events, which an outsider may find difficult to grasp. An outsider, however, may be permitted to ask questions of participants that an insider would be unable to ask because of their own or others' expectation, that they should know or have at least an idea of the answer. It is likely that a facilitator who is an outsider to the setting and/or organization could visit one setting to obtain background information. The information and interpretations obtained will of course be partial and incomplete, but could help inform the development of the training programme and give insights into the politics and culture of the organization at one local setting.

Facilitators coming from within the organization or home may feel that they do not need to get to know the setting and that Phases 1 and 2 of the training process are time-wasting exercises. I would argue strongly that this is not the case. Any view of the care setting will be partial, and insider knowledge that is taken for granted may obscure other views and opinions of the care setting. To take time to stand back from the impressions one has formed over time and look at the care setting using a different set of questions can be a highly illuminating process. Individuals may question what they are doing and why they are doing something on a regular or irregular basis – this is part of becoming a reflective practitioner. However, the processes suggested in Phases 1 and 2 involve looking at other peoples views and actions, which is something we may tend to overlook or not be given the opportunity to explore. Thus there are benefits to the observation process for any facilitator, whether they are an insider or outsider to the organization.

AUDIT

The word audit is associated with many types of investigations invoked by regulators, consumers, producers, citizens and states

(Power 1997). People are aware that audit is a way to explore accountability and in some way 'check up' on them. Thus it is hardly surprising that the word 'audit' can be a source of disquiet for staff. However, as care settings cater for vulnerable people it is appropriate that the care setting is open to scrutiny through audit, and it seems reasonable to investigate homes to ensure quality standards are maintained and if necessary improved. Individuals, however, may feel threatened by others (employees of the same organization or outsiders) asking questions and looking closely at their workplace and care practices. If the facilitator has begun to accumulate knowledge of the politics and culture of the organization they may be aware of the protocol surrounding such investigations and may have developed tactics to deal with the culture of the organization. However, individuals can easily obstruct audits, mislaying and/or preventing access to information requested in a way that the facilitator may not expect. In addition, the stance the facilitator adopts may influence the reception they receive. Forging good communication links at the outset may help; it can also help to be open about the purpose of the audit and what will be done with the information recorded. There may, however, be highly defensive people within the organization who will be threatened by the perceived intrusion of the facilitator into their workplace. It may be necessary to draw upon the knowledge, skills and position of managers at the higher organizational level or the owner of a private home for support. The facilitator may need to 'chase up' the individuals who are the holders of information required at regular intervals. Gaps in information given and the tactics individuals use to prevent the facilitator from gaining information are of course a source of insight into the culture of the care setting, and can provide the facilitator with knowledge upon which to base training exercises and which they can use to prepare themselves for possible difficult responses from participants. Of course, there will be individuals who are highly receptive and open to the audit process, particularly if they identified the training need to begin with and/or have a genuine desire to improve the service they provide.

There are many types of audit, but for the purposes of getting to know the care setting a structural audit complements observations and conversations. A structural audit gives the facilitator the opportunity to become familiar with the policies, procedures and philosophy or ethos of the care setting. There are many existing audits that could be used to evaluate the care setting. The Multiphasic Enviromental Assessment Procedure (MEAP) (Moos and Lemke 1992) is a popular tool in America, and the Royal College of Physicians in Britain have produced an extremely thorough assessment tool, the Continuous Assessment Review and Evaluation (CARE), which is appropriate for the British context (Hopkins, Brocklehurst and Dickinson 1992). Both the MEAP and CARE explore in detail the physical environments and facilities available in a setting. There are other audit tools that could be selected if the facilitator only wishes to get an idea of resident dependency levels; (Mini Mental State Examination) (MMSE) and the Revised Elderly Persons Disability Scale (REPDS) are two of many that are frequently used. These tools are not without their problems. The MMSE, for example, often causes distress to those who are asked questions they have difficulty answering, which begs the question of whether the insights gained warrant the distress caused to individuals? Organizations often have their own quality audits, which may be used or referred to if the facilitator wishes to look at the expected standards within a home and determine whether the home meets these. The facilitator should be clear about the purpose of using an audit tool, explore the information each tool is likely to yield and decide whether this information would be of benefit to the training programme. In addition, existing tools may be cumbersome and time- consuming, and if they do not collect information that is relevant to the project concerned, should be avoided. If this is the case it may be that there is a need for a new audit tool that meets the requirements of the overall training strategy of the organization or the dementia care training strategy. The facilitator or other people within the organization may be responsible for its design.

I found designing an audit tool to fit the requirements of a training project to be extremely valuable (Innes 1998). Factors such as staff and resident turnover provided insights into the stability of the workforce. If there is high staff turnover it is likely that staff may feel that they do not belong to a team. High staff turnover could indicate poor working conditions or dissatisfaction with the culture of the care setting, or could be an indication that there are more lucrative local job opportunities. High turnover of residents could alert the facilitator to potential feelings of bereavement and loss within the staff group. It may provide partial explanations if staff appear unwilling to engage in training that requires them to get to know the people they care for, which could lead to emotional attachments and then feelings of loss. Facilitators may also wish to explore the physical setting and the resources available to staff to help them with their work. In addition, the impact of the physical environment on resident mobility inside and outside the building can be examined, as can whether the environment provides stimulation and opportunities for residents to take part in activities and occupations they enjoy.

WORKING IN THE SETTING

It may be appropriate for the facilitator to work a couple of shifts within the setting to enable conversations, observations and collection of audit information to take place. If this is the case it is imperative that all staff are made aware of why the facilitator is working alongside them. It is important that reassurances are given that the facilitator is not a 'spy' who is going to check up on them and report back to management in a manner that is detrimental to the staff group. Working alongside staff may help the facilitator to gain credibility in the eyes of care staff, as the facilitator will demonstrate skills they also have and gain hands-on knowledge of the client group participants in the training programme work. Time constraints may prevent the facilitator from working alongside staff, as may the politics and dynamics of the organization. Observations and conversations may compensate for not being in a position to work alongside staff, while working alongside staff may negate the need to observe and talk at different times. The context within which the training takes place will influence the way(s) in which the facilitator gets to know the setting. Carrying training out 'blind', – that is with no knowledge of the staff group, client group, organization and care setting – could lead to a multitude of problems at a later date. Forewarned is forearmed, and therefore the knowledge gained in Phases 1 and 2 is of help to the facilitator. It enables the facilitator to develop a training programme that is relevant to the participants, alerts the facilitator to possible problems translating theory into practice, and prevents participants from having to engage with ideas that are irrelevant and/or unsuited to the realities of their practice (*see* Chapter 5).

SUGGESTED FURTHER READING

Chapter 6 in May's Social Research (1993) provides a readable account for those new to the idea of gaining information through conversations

Willcocks *et al.*(1987) book Private Lives in Public Places explores the idea of life in care homes being a different experience for staff and residents

Chapter 3

Designing the Training Programme

This third phase in the training process, designing the training programme, is often where facilitators begin. However, for this phase to be successful in that it produces a training programme that a) is likely to lead to the desired outcome of person-centred care for people with dementia and b) enables staff to develop reflective practitioner skills, the insights gained in Phases 1 and 2 are invaluable. Designing the training programme involves a number of considerations. Prior to the design of the training materials themselves or the structure of the sessions it is useful for the facilitator to consider learning theories. Insights gained from doing so can then be incorporated into the aims and objectives of the programme, the structure of the programme, the content of sessions and the exercises to be used within each training session.

LEARNING THEORIES

The teaching approach a facilitator will adopt is dependent upon the objectives of the programme. Do we want to equip staff with skills, provide knowledge, influence attitudes, or change the way staff work? A facilitator must consider such matters prior to designing the programme.

Theories of adult learning, termed andragogy by Knowles (1970), have led to wide recognition that adults as learners have special needs. Andragogy is built on four assumptions:

1.   Adults have a wealth of life experience to draw upon as a learning resource.

2.   Adults tend to have a problem-orientated approach to learning rather than the subject approach traditionally taken when teaching children (despite evidence that children do not necessarily respond well to this approach).

3.   An adult perceives their self as a self-directed human being.

4.   An adult's learning is orientated towards the task of fulfilling social roles.

The didactic 'chalk and talk' style often used in classrooms is not the most productive way for adults to learn, although people can enjoy this way of learning, particularly if the speaker is charismatic and the topic of real interest to the listeners. As adults come to the training programme with a wealth of experience and skills accumulated through life it is appropriate to draw upon the techniques of experiential and problem-based learning theories.

EXPERIENTIAL LEARNING

The theory of experiential learning, of which Knowles' (1970) theory of andragogy is a cornerstone, is essentially about enabling participants on a training programe to use their own experiences as a medium for insight and understanding. Kolb (1994) has built upon the theory of experiential learning by developing the idea of a learning cycle which begins and constantly returns to the individual's experiences. Thus, when an event is experienced the individual reflects on and learns from it, and when another experience occurs they will draw on prior experiences and reflections. Experiential learning techniques encourage participants on a training programme to draw upon and then reflect on their own experiences. For example, before carrying out life history work with residents, participants can be asked to reflect on their own life experiences by:

1. Thinking about five events that they would not want to forget and that they would like included in their own life history work.

2. Thinking of three objects they would like put in their own life history object box.

3. Thinking of things they would not want included in a life history book available for all staff to see.

The first two exercises can help participants draw upon their own life experiences (either on their own, in pairs or in small groups), which can be fed back to and discussed with the wider group. This enables the facilitator to highlight similarities between life events that the staff group have experienced such as marriage, childbirth and first job, achievements which may be unique but are still common ground that they share not only amongst themselves but also with people with dementia. The third exercise can help staff identify sensitive areas that life history work may uncover, and start a discussion on possible ways to deal with distress if it arises and how best to record the information.

PROBLEM-BASED LEARNING

Problem-based learning starts from the assumption that learning is effective when participants are given hypothetical examples (drawn from real life) to work through and 'solve' in the way they think best. This encourages participants to use the same techniques in their workplace (which many do already, thus validating this as an appropriate way in which to work and learn from experience). Therefore, staff could be given a short case study of a person with dementia, similar to the brief description of Mrs Stewart outlined below, that would provoke discussions on how to obtain the resident's consent to begin life history work and where to obtain background information.

Case Study

Mrs Stewart has lived at Greenacres for three months. She was admitted from hospital following a stroke which has left her temporarily in a wheelchair and apparently unable to communicate verbally. Staff were given no background information about Mrs Stewart on her admission. Mrs Stewart has had no visitors.

This is a very brief description but it is similar to the initial information staff often receive when a new resident enters a care home. It could be used as a starting point for individual work and group discussion on ways to find potential sources of information that would help staff care for Mrs Stewart.

STUDENT-CENTRED LEARNING

The government is currently advancing the need for lifelong learning to help the workforce keep up with a rapidly changing world. Lifelong learning starts from the premises that every situation encountered is a learning experience and that everyone has the potential to learn new skills and ideas throughout their lifespan. Thus the experiential and problem-solving approaches to teaching and learning can be utilized to help and encourage all workers to keep developing their abilities through experience and reflection.

It can be seen that a training programme utilizing theories of adult learning and experiential and problem-based training exercises is fundamentally a student-centred model of learning.

The students' experiences and ideas are at the centre of such a learning experience. At Bradford Dementia Group our starting point is the person-centred approach to the care of people with dementia; our training courses for staff extend this notion and are based upon a model of student-centred learning which places the student at the centre of the learning experience. The facilitator is not regarded as an expert, but more as a catalyst for student learning, and the assumption is that the trainer will also learn through facilitating the training programme.

There are three main elements to a student-centred model of learning:

1. The experience of students is of the utmost importance.

2. Training should enable participants to draw upon their experience, reflect and then work through exercises, which tend to be of a problem-solving nature.

3. People have many different learning styles, and training must encompass as many as possible to try to meet the style of the learner.

Individual training programmes will have various aims. If a student-centred model is adhered to, it is logical that an implicit aim of training is to develop practitioners who reflect on their experiences and learn from them in a process similar to that outlined by lifelong learning theorists.

REFLECTIVE PRACTITIONERS

Schons' work on reflective practice (1983; 1987) has particular relevance to student-centred learning programmes. If staff are to return to work and implement, for example, the skills learnt in theory and through problem-based and experiential exercises they are in essence reflecting on their learning and putting it into their practice. As Kitwood (1998) recently suggested, it is not the content of the training that is easy to transfer but the *process*. If training can begin to get participants to use processes that are amenable to transfer into practice there is an increased chance of the theory, or content, of training being transferred into the day-to-day practice of participants. In addition, the training may have begun or indeed be building upon previous training designed to encourage staff to become reflective practitioners. This is the concept I regard as central to training and the basis upon which to judge the success of a training programme (Phases 5 and 6 of the training process).

STRUCTURE OF THE PROGRAMME
Aims

With any training programme it is helpful for all concerned to know what exactly it is that the programme is aiming to achieve. If teachers and learners both know what is expected of them then it is more likely that they will be able to succeed. For example, the overall aim of a life-history training programme may be to introduce life-history work into the daily practice of the care setting

Objectives

Following on from the overall aim there may be a series of objectives such as:

1. For participants to be aware of the merits and difficulties of life-history work and the ways in which life-history material can be used and collected.

2. For staff to complete a life history with a resident of their choice.

3. For the information collected to be used in care planning.

PRACTICAL CONSIDERATIONS

There will be constraints placed on the facilitator which they may have little or no control over, such as the venue and the number of hours that the purchaser will fund or that the manager can persuade their staff to attend.

Venue

If the training programme is to be held in-house, it is important that the facilitator allows adequate time to set up and ensure that there are enough seats and tables, good lighting, ventilation and audibility, and teaching aids such as pens, flip charts and an overhead projector. Although these are basic and perhaps obvious considerations it can be easy to overlook circumstances that will not be conducive to learning and create a tense atmosphere

Timing

Timing issues include the length of each session within the programme and the number of sessions that make up the programme. In addition, the time of day at which the sessions are scheduled to take place requires consideration. Will staff rotas be flexible enough to meet the staffing needs of the setting but allow staff to attend, particularly night staff? It is likely that each session will need to be repeated at least twice to allow coverage of the work place, making allowances for days off and shift patterns.

It is also useful to consider the overall timing of the programme. For example, it may prove more difficult for management to arrange cover during holiday periods and therefore less staff may be able to attend the training. Also, certain times of year may be particularly busy for the care setting, such as Christmas preparations and annual quality inspections. There may be one-off events such as the restructuring or cutting back of the work force, or changes in shift patterns that could cause unrest and tension. If training is introduced at such times it could prove difficult for staff to attend and may be an irritant for staff at a time when they have additional tasks and/or stresses to cope with.

CONTENT

There are many stages involved in the design phase of a training programme. It is possible that the initial training steering or support group will have identified key areas that they wish to address through a training programme. When the facilitator is getting to know the setting further issues may arise that will inform the design of the training programme. The two areas may complement or conflict with one another. The group of people involved initially in the setting up of a training strategy may need to consult further in order to decide on the course of action to be taken.

Those purchasing the training may have no idea what they want other than training in 'dementia care', thus the 'getting to know the setting' phase will be vital for the facilitator, staff and persons with dementia. The facilitator who takes a pre-designed programme to a setting is likely to encounter numerous problems. Problems may not be evident at the delivery stage, but when it comes to translating the theory into practice, lack of knowledge of the context in which it is hoped that training will have an effect could be the downfall of an otherwise theoretically sound training programme.

If the manager of a setting has identified a need for training in a particular area it is important that the facilitator liaises with the manager to clarify the purpose of the training and what may reasonably be attainable within any time and resource constraints. There may be disagreements as to what is required after the facilitator has completed the 'getting to know the setting' phase, which must be discussed and resolved in a mutually agreeable way.

If the original phase of 'getting started' has gone well (i.e. the facilitator has gained knowledge and insight into the organization and established good channels of communication) any subsequent discussions about content should be easier. There is of course the possibility that the facilitator will be given a free rein to design the programme as they see fit based on their evaluation of the setting, but even then it is useful for the facilitator to inform other key players about their decisions.

A variety of examples will be used to illustrate key issues for consideration when devising a training programme designed to help staff work towards the person-centred approach to care. If person-centred care is to become a reality, a good starting point is for care staff to build up a knowledge bank for each resident in their care. This would cover not only residents' current likes and dislikes and physical care needs but also knowledge of their pasts. What were their achievements? What did they enjoy? What did they do in their spare time? Did they work? The past and its effect on the present can then perhaps be better understood. (For a readable introduction to life-history work see Charlie Murphy's *It Started With a Seashell* (1994)). Care staff often have detailed knowledge of those they care for, but this is not always used directly to inform the care process. Staff may have information on some residents but not others, and may be unsure about where to obtain the information.

If the programme is designed to encourage staff to collect and use life-history information with the residents in their care, the training must address the rationale for doing life-history work, who will benefit (e.g. staff, residents, relatives) and in what ways. Discussion of possible sources of information may help. Such sources could be:

- the resident themselves
- relatives and friends of the person with dementia
- other staff
- if the resident has had one prior to admission, a CPN (Community Psychiatric Nurse) or social worker, who may be willing to help

- the resident's GP, who may be willing to fill in some gaps
- neighbours
- any group that the resident belonged to at one time
- church congregations, if the resident previously attended a church.

The list could go on. It may aid staff to be made aware that they may be given two or more versions of the same events, depending on who provides the information. Although it may be tempting for staff to see family members' versions as the 'truth', it is likely that the person themselves will remember details that have meaning and significance to them, and this is their 'truth'. Multiple accounts of an event can be very enlightening on how family members perceive their relative and also how the resident remembers their family and their place within it. This may help staff to understand family members' distress at their mother or father's decline in cognitive abilities.

In addition, ways in which the life-history material can be recorded and brought together can be discussed and debated. For example, loose ring binders could be used, objects could be placed in a memory box, care plans could be developed to contain more detailed life history information than is normally the case. The ethics of gathering material and how to obtain the resident's consent need to be discussed. Is it acceptable to record information without the person's consent? Should family members be consulted? Does the assent of family members to life-history work override the resident's objections? Discussions such as these may stimulate interest in life-history work and alert staff to potential difficulties and issues they may have to address when they begin life-history work. Key information to be included in a life- history can be discussed and debated. Kitwood and Bredin's *Person to Person: A Guide to the Care of those with Failing Mental Powers* (1992a, p.15)) contains a list of highly-relevant questions to ask when doing life history work. What is the person's family background? What do they value? What are their religious beliefs? If the theory behind life-history work is to be put into practice, staff must begin *doing* life history work. It is more likely to be successful if staff choose a person they would like to work with, perhaps someone they are key worker for. Any potential difficulties and problems staff identify initially can be considered within the training sessions, as can ways to overcome them.

The above is an example of what might be included either in a programme focusing only on life-history work or as a part of a wider programme addressing other key issues in dementia care such as the environment, care planning, risk-taking, and choice and communication. (This list is a suggestion – there are many other areas that may be identified as useful for a particular setting or organization.)

EXERCISES

If the training programme adheres to a student-centred model then exercises of a problem-solving nature are appropriate, as are exercises which draw upon the participants' experiences.

The work of Honey and Mumford (1982) has led to widespread recognition that different people have different learning styles. They suggest that reflectors, theorists, pragmatists and activists are the principle types of learner, although of course there may be individuals who will have two or more of the suggested learning styles. It is important that the facilitator considers the different ways in which participants on the training programme may learn, and that they design or use exercises that incorporate more than one particular learning style in order to try to avoid preventing individuals from learning in the way that they prefer. It may be that working in small groups will be enjoyed by most and individual work by fewer people, but it is important to provide a mix of types of exercise so as to enable participants to experience different ways of working and learning and also to meet their needs. Pair work is another option, as is the whole group participating in, for example, a brainstorming session. There may be times when the facilitator must talk in the manner associated with lectures. If this is the case then talks should be interspersed with group participation, as continual listening offers no opportunities to share thoughts, ideas and experiences, is not a very pleasant experience and does not place the student at the centre of the learning experience.

Designing training exercises can be difficult at first, and it is only through use that any flaws in exercises become evident. There are, however, sources that would-be facilitators can draw upon. Weiner (1997), for example, is a good source of creative training ideas and the dementia-specific training pack by Loveday, Kitwood and Bowe (1998) provides many exercises that facilitators can draw upon and use in their training programmes. For the facilitator and participants to engage fully with the materials and give them reality, it is helpful if the facilitator can develop scenarios and vignettes based on their own experience. These can then be developed into a problem-solving exercise and the real outcome compared to that suggested by the participants. It is important to include both 'good' and 'bad' outcomes within the examples so as to allow participants to develop ideas that could have led to better outcomes for the residents and staff members concerned. Names of individuals and places used in training exercises should be changed so as to maintain their anonymity.

The following examples of short vignettes drawn from my experience have lead to discussions, sometimes heated, within training sessions on a number of issues. Any facilitator can use this format by including examples from their own experience, but their vignettes should still cover the same broad issues.

1. Jimmy has only been at Acorn Drive for two weeks. His nephew told staff that his uncle was a very active man who worked as a bus driver for the last 20 years of his working life. Staff are finding it very difficult to cope with Jimmy 'wandering' and going out onto the main road and getting on any bus that passes by. It is decided to put Jimmy on medication that will 'calm him down'.

This example encourages staff to think about three broad issues:

   (a) the appropriateness of medication as a form of restraint.

   (b) their own attitudes and beliefs about risk-taking and their often conflicting roles of defending residents' rights but minimizing risk.

   (c) why the person is behaving in such a way and what might be the underlying issues, e.g. boredom, disorientation.

2. Arthur is a very sociable man. One day he was walking in the lounge with Sandra, a care assistant, when suddenly he pulled her very close to himself and tried to kiss her.

This example encourages staff to consider:

   (a) the reason(s) Arthur may have behaved in such a way.

   (b) similar situations they have found themselves in and how they reacted.

   (c) possible ways to respond to situations in which they may feel uncomfortable.

ANOTHER OBJECTIVE – TEAM BUILDING?

The implicit or explicit purpose of training may be to promote team building and group working. If exercises can help staff to value one another and work together rather than feel like they work in isolation from one another, it is likely that the training will be of benefit to participants. It has been suggested that team problem-solving exercises can validate staff feelings of frustration with the constraints they operate under and help to create a sense of co-operation and mutual support, which could in turn lead to staff being more open to change (Frazier and Sherlock 1994, p.121). Therefore, training that is seeking to change or develop the way in which staff work may be more effective if team building is integral to the content of the programme.

SUGGESTED FURTHER READING

Rogers (1986) and Cross (1981), provide useful starting points for those who are unfamiliar with the notion of adult learning and adult learning theories.

Chapter 4

Delivering the Training Programme

If the facilitator has got to know the setting and has carefully planned the structure and content of the training, then necessary conditions for the successful delivery of training have been considered. These necessary conditions are not, however, always sufficient to guarantee successful training sessions. This chapter outlines two broad areas that a facilitator may find useful to consider and, if possible, prepare for before and during the delivery of the training. The first area a facilitator may need to consider and devise strategies for dealing with is *group dynamics*. It should be remembered that the culture of the workplace, identified during Phases 1 and 2 of the training process, can have an effect on the dynamics within the training sessions and influence the possibility of participants developing ideas to use in their practice. However, the group dynamics within individual training sessions can have a life of their own and may contribute to a positive environment that is conducive to learning or create a tense, stifling atmosphere. The second area a facilitator needs to consider is that there are a number of personal skills and/or qualities that they may need to draw upon to ensure that the training sessions go smoothly and, develop strategies to cope with difficulties should they arise.

GROUP DYNAMICS

There can be a number of underlying tensions to which the training programme facilitator needs to be sensitive. There are many benefits of having all members of a staff team participate in a training programme. The sharing of knowledge and experience can provoke lively discussion and debate. Senior staff may enable and encourage staff to air their opinions and share their experiences. For example:

Case Study

Paul has been the manager of Daisy House Residential Home for two years. He is enthusiastic about the training programme and glad that staff will learn together, and hopes that in the process the staff group will 'gel' together. During training sessions he encourages staff to share their experiences of care work and the client group. Paul admits to staff that he doesn't always have the answers and that the direct 'hands on' work of other members of the staff group means that they will often have useful ideas. Staff appear happy to contribute and often challenge Paul's ideas.

However, the presence of senior staff within a training session may inhibit junior members of staff:

Case Study

Sylvia has been the manager of Acorn Drive Residential Care Home for four years. She has attended a number of training courses for managers over the same period of time. Sylvia agreed to attend the training sessions with the senior team within the home (assistant

---

Case Study (continued)

managers and senior care assistants) and all other members of staff, including care assistants, domestics, catering staff and the maintenance person. During the course of a training session Sylvia is the first to contribute to brainstorming sessions and nominates herself as spokesperson for small-group work. She becomes angry with staff who offer a different perspective to her own. Staff have begun to wait until she offers her opinion and are apprehensive about sharing alternative viewpoints.

Senior staff may dominate discussions and/or dismiss the contributions of junior staff. For example:

Case Study

Mavis is an assistant manager at the Beeches Nursing Home. She is a Registered Mental Nurse. Mavis questioned why she should attend a training programme with care assistants who had not received the nursing training she had. After discussion of the benefits of all staff learning together and sharing skills and knowledge Mavis agreed to attend. During the training Mavis sits at the back of the room, arms folded, looking out of the window. She does not contribute any ideas of her own but from time to time makes comments such as 'That's obvious', 'I know this already' or 'These are old ideas'.

Participants in the training session may use other forms of power to dominate or intimidate other participants. For example, male members of staff may use their gender to exert influence over the discussion, or older people may use their longer length of service as a way of overriding the opinions of younger staff. For example:

Case Study

During a discussion about activities Pam suggests that it would be good for a male resident, Jim, who used to be a baker, to join in baking sessions. Derek tells Pam to stick to what she knows as a woman. He says that as a man he knows what male residents will enjoy doing and that she should leave men to do men's work.

Case Study

Julie has worked as a care assistant at The Poplars for two months. She was employed following a successful voluntary work-experience placement which was organised by her school. Julie questions the ways in which staff currently work and offers new alternatives. Jean, who has been a care assistant for 20 years, the last four at the Poplars, tells Julie 'You should learn to work the way we do, we've been doing it for years, we don't need you to tell us what to do.'

There may be members of staff who have had romantic encounters that have ended, or staff who were friends out of work but have fallen out. Factors such as these can influence how the group will work together within a training session. There may have been arguments between staff prior to coming to the training. For example:

Case Study

During a training session Alice and Beth, who both work the night shift, refuse to work together in the same small group. They then begin to make critical comments on each other's ideas. Beth begins to question Alice's commitment to her work. The facilitator intervenes and it emerges that Alice often finds it difficult to find childcare during training events and staff meetings. The previous day she had been unable to find a childminder and could not to attend a staff meeting. She has, however, made arrangements so as to enable her to attend the training session. Beth is annoyed that Alice has not made time to attend both the staff meeting and the training.

In addition, staff may feel that the training is inappropriate for them and that they have been coerced into attending; if any preparatory materials have not been evenly distributed, some may have no idea what the training is about; and long-serving members of staff may feel that they have nothing to learn because they've heard or done it all before. There are countless scenarios that could have an impact on the dynamics of the group. Also, a group who worked well together one week may be antagonistic towards one another the following week. The facilitator must therefore be constantly alert to changes in group dynamics.

GROUND RULES

Many teachers and trainers in all areas develop sets of ground rules at the outset of their training programmes. Setting ground rules for the training programme may prevent some of the potential difficulties outlined above. Some trainers have a predetermined list of ground rules and may or may not give participants the chance to add to or amend these in line with their own perceptions of how the training can go well. A list of possible ground rules is suggested in the box below; however, ground rules tend to work best when the participants themselves agree and develop their own. This can be a beneficial warm-up exercise, and is particularly useful if participants do not know one another well. By setting their own ground rules participants can begin to see what others expect of them in the training sessions. This also applies to staff who do know one another well but who are used to, for example, supervising or being supervised. Setting ground rules can establish a climate of equality, at least within the training context, as participants agree that everyone should be given a fair hearing, and a chance to speak, that differences of opinion will be respected, and that the group will not operate on the basis of different levels of power and status within the workplace.

Ground Rules

1. Listening
Everyone in the group will try to give their full attention to the person who is speaking.

2. Confidentiality
Everyone in the group has a responsibility not to disclose information discussed in the training sessions that could identify individuals and breach client confidentiality.

---

3. Respecting differences

Everyone is different and because of this members of the group may have different views and opinions on certain issues. Group members will try to avoid judging others ('You should not do that/think that') but will explain if they disagree or are worried by the opinion voiced by another participant. Respecting differences does not mean that group members have to agree with one another about everything.

4. Expressing feelings

Care work can lead to strong feelings and attachments to clients. Training may bring out these feelings and group members will try and support one another.

5. Giving each individual participant equal time to talk

Participants will try not to 'hog' discussion times. Everyone in the group has had experiences from which others can learn.

6. Each individual has a responsibility to participate.

If individuals have something to say or share but feel shy or uncomfortable, for example, in large groups, they can share their views in pairs or small-group work for someone else to feed back to the wider group.

The facilitator may suggest that the group reviews the ground rules at the end of a session. If participants feel that they have not been treated well by others in the group this could be an explosive exercise. However, reviewing ground rules does offer participants the opportunity to engage with and reflect on their own and others' actions within the training session. This process may be of use to staff who do not tend to reflect on their own or others' practice in the course of their work. Reflecting on the training may provides the impetus for reflection to be introduced into day-to-day work practices.

Ground rules are not the only way in which the facilitator can work with existing group dynamics and help change them. The facilitator can also draw upon a number of personal skills and qualities that help in the delivery of the training programme.

SKILLS/QUALITIES THAT THE TRAINER MAY NEED TO CALL UPON

Loveday, Kitwood and Bredin (1998) suggest that the key qualities of a good facilitator are similar to the qualities required of a good care worker (p.30). If a facilitator can empathize with the problems participants face in their day-to-day work and the difficulties they have in trying to incorporate the ideas generated during training into their practice, there is an increased likelihood that the facilitator will be able to facilitate discussions in which participants feel that it is safe to be open about the problems they face. Another similarity is communication. A care worker needs to be creative when trying to maintain communication with a person who is apparently losing their ability to communicate in conventional ways. Facilitators also need to find ways to communicate with participants, perhaps finding alternative ways to demonstrate ideas and picking up on the non-verbal signs of participants, which may indicate when they are uncomfortable with ideas or are finding it difficult to enter discussions.

There are times when training sessions do not go as expected, when other issues enter the time set aside for training. Weiner (1997) suggests that when the session encounters problems 'team doctoring' may be required to attend to the problem and to move things on.

Case Study

Cliff View Nursing Home is in the process of changing the shift patterns of care assistants. This involves all staff working alternate weekends. A number of staff are angry about this decision as previously they did not work at weekends or only one weekend a month. Staff who had been employed solely for weekend shifts have been given the option of redundancy or integration within the new shift patterns.

If members of staff are about to undergo changes such as a reworking of shift patterns, they may feel unsettled and unhappy. It may be that the training session is the only place where staff are together as a group and therefore able to discuss how the changes may affect them and how they feel about this. It is likely that the facilitator will need to give staff time to discuss the issues that are bothering them, enabling (in theory) the group to move on.

Thus, if events emerge within the training sessions that are outside the facilitator's control and lead to a breakdown in participation, the facilitator must take stock and explore the available options. These are:

1. To give participants the time to air their concerns.

2. To allocate part of the session to the issues at the forefront of participants' minds.

3. To postpone the session until a later date.

The approach the facilitator takes will be dependent on circumstances, and thus the facilitator needs to be sensitive to situations, and flexible and responsive to the feelings of participants, skills care workers also often need to draw upon.

The following seven skills/qualities are among many that facilitators may need to develop to enable them to cope with the difficulties they encounter when facilitating group training

1. Organizational skills

The facilitator of a training programme needs to draw upon many organizational skills, before, during and after a training session. Prior to a session the facilitator has a great deal to organize. For example, handouts need to be typed and copied. Course materials need to be checked and copied. Before the handouts can be copied, the number of participants needs to be established. The venue needs to be organized and the facilitator has to check whether any of the necessary equipment (e.g. flip chart or overhead projector) is available. During the session the facilitator has to manage the time participants spend on exercises, discussion and breaks. In addition, the facilitator may have to help participants organize themselves into working groups, and once in the groups guide them through the relevant issues. After a training session or training programme the facilitator has to think about how they can develop the course for future use and, perhaps, organize for the distribution, collection and analysis of course feedback forms.

2. Mediating skills

The facilitator may need to draw upon these interpersonal skills and abilities throughout the training, particularly if the participants' debate slides into open warfare. There are various strategies for diffusing heated debates. For example, the facilitator may intervene by saying:

- 'Let's slow down a moment.'

- 'There seem to be a number of different opinions. Let's think these through and see what we can agree on.'

- 'We're not getting anywhere with this discussion. Those who want to continue with it can do so later. We'll move on now to another topic.'

This tactic does not need to be used every time an argument develops: it is often useful to let the debate flow, as lively discussions can often ensue. It is, however, important to intervene if individuals begin to attack one another.

3. Team-building

Team-building skills are often necessary, especially when staff are coming from different settings and do not know one another, or with a staff team who work in a hierarchical way which does not allow staff at the lower end of the hierarchy to have their say. If the facilitator is aware of a hierarchy within the workplace (as a result of the 'getting to know the setting' phase of the process) then the following exercise may form a useful basis for getting participants to value one another.

Case Study

Divide the group into pairs (if possible, mix nurses and care assistants, senior staff and junior staff together). Each person is given five minutes to tell the other something, that they value in the other person at work, something that they think the other person is good at. The group then reconvenes and each pair tells the rest of the group what they like about the way the other person works.

For staff who are coming together from different workplaces it is often useful to again divide the group into pairs and ask them to interview each other on a topic of their choice, e.g. family or favourite holiday destination. The group can then reconvene and each person can share the recently acquired information (with the other person's permission) with the whole group.

4. Patience/tolerance

This applies particularly to different views and opinions expressed within training sessions, some of which may be anathema to other participants and/or the facilitator. Problems may arise, for example, if the facilitator is promoting the person-centred approach to care and there are participants who continually stress that the 'dementia' is a barrier to this approach. Participants from minority ethnic groups may have to endure other participants' 'culture blaming' opinions about problems that these groups encounter. It may take time and patience to challenge such opinions and tolerance may not be an option if, for example, blatantly racist views are expressed.

5. A sense of humour

This helps when things go wrong or not to plan and when mistakes are made. Barriers can often be broken down if humour is introduced to the training session and if the facilitator can laugh at their own mistakes and difficulties. In my experience, having problems setting up a flip chart or overhead projector often leads to laughter amongst participants.

6. Perceptiveness

It is important to be sensitive to changes in the mood of the group and/or of individuals within it. Indications of this are:

- Several conversations taking place simultaneously.

- Ideas of individuals or small groups being attacked before they have been fully expressed.

- Excessive 'nit-picking'.

- Participants taking sides or ganging up on one individual.

The facilitator may then intervene or change tack. Calling a short break can also 'break' the atmosphere.

7. Empathy

If the facilitator can demonstrate an understanding of the stresses and satisfactions staff encounter in the course of their day-to-day work and any difficulties they may have with the training materials it is likely that participants will respond more positively to the training. There is a greater possibility that this will be achieved if the facilitator has successfully got to know the setting during Phase 2 of the training process.

In addition, the facilitator needs to be knowledgeable about the subject area. If the facilitator does not keep abreast with developments in the field and remain open to alternative views then it is likely that will be problems when delivering training materials. If the training diverges from the set topic area to an area that the facilitator is not familiar with, then it is perfectly acceptable and appropriate for the facilitator to admit that there are gaps in their knowledge base. This adds to the climate of equality that the ground rules may have established.

Chapter 5

Turning Training into Practice

'It's very interesting but not actually relevant to my work.'

The above comment about training sessions is one that many trainers, facilitators and participants may have heard on numerous occasions. This can create a real problem for facilitators: how can training be constructed so as to be not only relevant to staff but possible to put into practice? Two principal tactics that are fairly easy to pursue are assessment and action planning.

ASSESSMENT

The first tactic that can be used to ensure that training will have an impact on practice is that of incorporating an assessment into the training programme. One of the key tools care staff often use when working with people with dementia is a care plan. Traditional care plans often focus on physical care needs, and emphasize what the person can no longer do and needs help with rather than what the person can do and what assistance they may require to do so. If the training has emphasized the need for person-centred care then it would be appropriate to set an assessment in which participants write a section of a care plan focusing on the social and psychological needs and well-being of a person of their choice with dementia.

Participants should be given clear guidelines on how to complete the assessment. A guide is suggested below.

Care plan assessment

For this piece of work you will be able to draw upon topics covered during the training (programme). The care plan should begin with a short paragraph giving details about the person. This should be written in a way that emphasizes what the person can do – their strengths and achievements. You should also include a short statement on the person's needs and current state of well-being. Remember to broaden the focus from physical care needs to social needs.

Each of the following topics should be included:

- risk-taking

- rights

- responsibilities

- choice

- the environment

- activities.

Draw upon everything you have learnt from the training and try to relate it to any information you have about the person for whom you are writing the care plan. Bear in mind the following points:

- The care plan should be goal-orientated rather than task-orientated; the aim is to achieve positive changes in the person's well-being rather than just to carry out routine tasks.

- The care plan should take account of the person's strengths and abilities rather than just their needs and deficiencies.

- The care plan should take account of the person's own interests and opinions wherever possible.

Assessment Criteria

- Clear, well-organized presentation, showing attention to the instructions given above.

- The ability to recognize the needs and abilities of the person with dementia.

- Evidence of a positive, goal-orientated approach to care planning.

A suggested format sheet can be given to complement the written instructions:

Background Paragraph:

Goal	Plan(s)
1.	
2.	
3.	
4.	

Figure 5.1 Care plan assessment format sheet

Assessments can be written or oral and will vary according to what is being assessed. If a course has been concerned with providing participants with knowledge then a simple series of questions can be put together. For example:

1. Open-ended questions

- What do you consider to be key aspects of the person-centred approach to care? Give three examples.

- Why is it important to have life-history information for each person with dementia?

2. Multiple-choice questions

The most common form of dementia is

(a)   Alzheimer's Disease

(b)   Vascular dementia

(c)   Korsakoff's disease

(d)   Pick's disease.

3. Simple true-or-false questions (these can be used when it is too difficult to come up with more than two plausible answers)

There is no known cure for dementia. True/False

If the course has been concerned with equipping staff with skills, for example using new hoists, then it is reasonable to assess competence by observing the member of staff demonstrating on another participant in the first instance and then on a resident. (There are many issues to be considered when assessing practice. Interested readers may wish to refer to the English National Board publication *Researching Professional Education: Levels of Achievement: A review of the Assessment of Practice* (Gerrish,

McManus and Ashworth 1997) for a thorough introduction to recent developments in the nursing field.)

It can be difficult to assess whether a training programme has had an effect on participants' attitudes. Questionnaires can be used at the beginning and end of a training programme to try to ascertain whether there have been any shifts in outlook. However, it is notoriously difficult to assess attitudes through questionnaires (for a full discussion see Oppenheim 1966). Even if another method, such as DCM, is used to establish whether person-centred responses are more prevalent, it would be difficult to judge whether it is only behaviour that has changed (perhaps because the participants are being observed) or whether the underlying thought processes behind actions and behaviour have actually altered. People are capable of doing one thing but thinking another.

It will take time to ascertain whether changes brought about within the culture of a care setting or organization are long-lasting. A recent study (Moniz-Cooke et al. 1998) found that changes in practice begun by a training programme had not been sustained over the following year. They suggest that regular supervision may have helped to support staff in their endeavors to work in a different way and that the home environment may also be an important determinant of the success of a training programme. The training may have aimed to establish good team working, and although this may be achieved in the short term, the pressures of the work, staff shortages and staff and resident turnover are likely to have an effect on group dynamics and working relationships. I would suggest that if the facilitator has committed time and effort to the 'getting to know the setting' phase and considered the politics of the organization (as outlined in chapter 1 above) then there should, in theory, be an increased chance of a successful and effective training prog-ramme, as factors such as a lack of supervision or effective working relationships would have been identified and strategies devised to deal with these issues.

ACTION PLANS

Facilitating the development of staff action plans is another possible way of turning learning into practice and at the same time enabling and empowering staff to put forward their ideas for debate and implementation in their work place. Action plans can take several forms:

- At a very basic individual level, staff can be asked to write down a *personal pledge* to share with others in the group. When an individual makes a personal pledge they state their commitment to an idea that they can take away from the training session and attempt to incorporate into their practice. For example, following a session on risk-taking, staff may pledge to try to give residents freedom and choice by allowing them to go into the garden unattended or finding ways to enable residents to smoke unsupervised.

- Action plans can take on the ideas of the whole group. Each participant can be asked to identify one thing that, as a result of the training programme, they would like to see more of, less of or introduced into the care setting. (For example, in relation to the environment.) Individuals' ideas can be put up on the wall and grouped into broad areas. After consideration of the environment some participants may have focused on the garden or outside areas, others on communal inside areas and others on staff areas. Individuals can then be grouped together to discuss which of the similar ideas they would like to focus on. The benefits of and reasons for proposing a certain action can be discussed, highlighting for themselves and others the implications of any proposed actions in terms of resources and practical support from other staff, residents, relatives etc. Examples of proposed actions are outlined below:

Table 5.1 'Environment' Related Proposals

Proposed Action	Benefits/reasons	Implications
To buy bird tables, nut bags and growbags containing tomato plants	1. Would encourage birds to come into the garden. This would give residents the opportunity to look for different kinds of birds 2. Residents could be taken into the garden to fill nut bags and put food on the table and hence would give them something to do	• the cost of the bird table • paying for nuts • low outlay costs • low running costs, e.g. dry bread could be used.
To make upstairs lounge into an activities room	1. Large room 2. Sink and water available for painting etc. 3. Toilets close by	• low cost.
Clients to have their own window boxes	1. Would provide clients with something to look at and show to their family and friends 2. Creates a good impression for visitors 3. May give residents a sense of achievement	• money for equipment • may give the home a better image • staff could perhaps bring in seeds/bulbs from own gardens.
Improve garden and access to garden areas	1. Could have vegetable plot for residents to use 2. Would be a pleasant area for residents to spend some time 3. More flowers/garden furniture and a bird table would be stimulating for residents	• cost of plot, seeds, any furniture • would need advice on layout • gardener?
Music/TV/ video room for residents who enjoy watching in quiet surroundings	1) Those who do not want to watch TV have greater choice 2) Happier residents 3) Relaxed atmosphere 4) Reduces stress levels for all staff	• loss of revenue from room.

Each small group's proposal can be passed around the other groups for comments to be added, creating the sense of a 'group' effort. Each group's proposed action can be put together into one document, made available to all staff and presented to the person(s) staff think will be most influential in getting their ideas put into practice (most probably management at home and possibly organization level).

It may be that the action plans that staff develop are so comprehensive that it will be necessary to have follow-up training sessions to help staff prioritize their ideas and think through any further implications. For their action plans to be successful staff will need the backing of many people; those who the proposed actions will impact upon, those who have the power within the care setting to make things happen and, if additional resources are required, possibly management at the overall organizational level. It is useful to consider possible obstacles to the implementation of staff care-plan ideas and proposed actions. Obstacles can come from within the care setting itself and are thus shaped by *internal forces*, or from outside the care setting and are thus shaped by *external forces*.

OBSTACLES TO IMPLEMENTATION

1. Internal forces

(a) Staff turnover

Staff turnover can have potentially damaging effects on the implementation of the ideas of training participants. New staff may not be committed to the ideas within the action plan (this is highly probable given that they had no involvement in formulating them), and it is likely that there may be opposition or apathy. New staff may be used to working in ways that are different to those established in the organization itself and those suggested within the training programme. However, if new staff receive a thorough induction, the action plans are explained to them and they are given the opportunity to add their own ideas there is an increased likelihood that new staff will take 'ownership' of the action plan.

(b) Resident turnover

The death of residents or the loss of those who are moved on to nursing homes from residential homes or to hospital from nursing homes can be traumatic events for staff and residents. The circumstances surrounding the departure of a resident may be unusual and upsetting, and if staff have established good relationships with such residents then they can be left with a sense of loss and grief that may be unacknowledged within a care setting. Low staff morale may develop, resulting in new ideas and enthusiasm being lost. A sensitive and aware management team can help to address this by offering support to staff and helping to keep the action plan on track.

(c) Staff burn-out and illness

This often occurs when there are staff shortages and poor working conditions but can occur at times of change such as the restructuring of the workforce, times of high resident or staff turnover and, often, at holiday times, when staff work longer hours to cover for workmates. There has been much work on burn-out and staff distress (McCrane, Lambert and Lambert 1987; Cohen-Mansfield 1989). Care work is by its very nature stressful: care staff encounter death, illness and people who may be emotionally demanding. These 'stressors' are part and parcel of care work and impossible to avoid. McCrane *et al.* suggest that there are organizational interventions such as increasing staffing levels and providing staff with support that may help reduce stressors that appear to contribute to burn-out.

(d) Support structures

The issue of support structures is elaborated in relation to dementia care workers by Kitwood and Woods (1996). They argue that it is necessary to design a good support structure for staff when considering a development strategy for a new home. Supervision and induction systems are, however, important not only to new homes but also to existing homes. If staff do not receive an adequate induction to their workplace, their particular role within it and its underlying philosophy of care practice then it will be a difficult task to integrate new members of staff into the staff team. Similarly, if staff do not receive regular feedback on their performance and help in identifying their development needs through formal and/or informal supervision it is likely that staff may become demoralized and 'stuck' in a particular way of working. The absence of support mechanisms such as supervision, communication procedures and training for staff can contribute towards apathy, discontent, and a general lack of awareness of what is going on within the care setting and/or the organization. This may contribute to staff finding it difficult to implement ideas discussed within training into their daily practice. It is logical that if staff feel unsupported and are unaware of the philosophy or approaches which the organization is supporting there will be a mismatch between the official line and actual practice. If support systems are in place it is likely that staff will be committed to the care setting and the morale of the staff group will be high.

(e) Resistance to change

If the training is suggesting changes to the ways in which people work there can be many sources of resistance. Amongst these are:

- *Individuals.* There may be members of the staff group who oppose the ideas generated by the training programme. It may be that the training threatens their power base. For example, if, traditionally, it is the manager of a home who generates new ideas and the training invites all staff to contribute to this process, the way in which members of the staff group relate to one another changes. Care staff may be empowered by this change, as they are given the opportunity to voice their opinions. However, the manager may feel undermined and/or threatened, as s/he is no longer the only source of ideas. Furthermore, existing practices, which were probably the original ideas of the manager, may be challenged. In addition, the training may promote ideas which are contrary to deep-rooted practices and care traditions, or an individual may like the way they do things now and simply have no desire to try out new ideas.

- *Groups.* There may be considerable group inertia and the force of habit may be difficult to overcome. In addition, there may be pressure on individuals from groups within the care setting whose members do not want to change the way they work Occupational groups within the setting may be resistant to change if their power bases or claims to aspects of the work are threatened. For example, nurses may be reluctant to allow care assistants to carry out traditional 'nursing' tasks, or occupational therapists may be reluctant to allow anyone else to arrange recreational activities.

- *Management* (individuals or the team). Members of the management team may perceive that any change may challenge or threaten the existing power structure. If management perceives change as leading to some of its power going to other groups it could use its existing power to resist any suggested changes.

2. External forces

(a) New policies

New policies that appear to run counter to the messages of training may be introduced, thus confusing staff as to what it is that they should be trying to achieve. New policies may outline steps that staff must take immediately within their work, thus taking precedence over practices established by the training programme.

(b) New procedures

The introduction of new procedures from within the organization or from other external bodies such as purchasers of beds may result in new paperwork and reorganization, again taking precedence over the implementation of training ideas or simply giving staff no time to do anything else.

(c) Restructuring of the staff group

Restructuring of staff and/or streamlining of organizations can result in redundancies, which create discord. New job roles or job descriptions can cause friction and confusion as staff try to work in new positions, possibly with new staff or staff who have been promoted or demoted, resulting in new dynamics between staff in the care setting. Delays in restructuring, once announced, can cause further discord as staff are left 'hanging', not knowing what the restructuring will mean for them.

(d) Changes in the funding/finance of a setting

Financial changes can lead to a sense of disquiet if staff are aware that funding is an issue that could have repercussions on their own job security. In addition, new policies and procedures may take effect as funding sources change.

WHAT HELPS TO OVERCOME OBSTACLES?

One possible block to staff implementation of ideas discussed within training sessions is staff burn-out. If staff burn-out can be prevented or reduced, the workplace is likely not only to be one that is conducive to staff learning but one that encourages staff to act upon their learning. Aronson (1994) suggests that training and skills development is necessary to help reduce or prevent staff burnout (p.41). In addition, she suggests that the encouragement of innovation, supervisory leadership, administrative support and availability of information can all help to reduce staff burn-out and stress. Therefore, training may help to reduce or prevent staff burn-out, but other factors also need to be considered.

The recruitment process for new staff is a vital consideration. If staff who do not believe in the organization's philosophy of care are recruited, it is likely that any training and development work the organization initiates will not have the desired effect. Kitwood and Woods (1996) regard the selection of senior staff and care assistants as essential to the strategy of a care setting, they suggest that the job specification for any level of care position should emphasize the attitudes required to deliver person- centred care (pp.8–10). At interview, applicants can be asked to describe good and bad practice on the basis of their own experiences. Kitwood and Woods suggest that previous experience of caring, in any context, should be considered as a relevant qualification. Frazier and Sherlock (1994) suggest similar key criteria for working with people with dementia: personal warmth, good communication skills, the ability to work as part of a team, initiative and creativity (p.111). In addition, they suggest that staff need to be receptive to supervision and that, if possible, they should have had prior experience of working with people with dementia and understand the 'symptomatology/behavioural manifestations of dementia'. These two criteria contradict the view of Kitwood and Woods (1996) that previous experience and knowledge of dementia are not necessarily important, but a view that is logical, because if the applicant shares the attitudes and values of the person-centred approach to care (attitudes and values that are readily transferable to the care setting) it is likely that training can help them to gain the specific knowledge of dementia required for their work. Current staff groups may not have been recruited along the lines suggested above, and therefore there may be individuals attending the training programme who it will be difficult for the facilitator to win over. It may be necessary to provide individuals with supervision and support to encourage them to go through an appropriate and thorough personal development process.

In the absence of the above factors, which may help to overcome obstacles, there are interim measures that may aid the implementation of the ideas generated through training. The initial steering or support group, set up during Phase 1 of the training process to introduce the training programme to a care setting, may be in a position to manage individuals who are resistant to the philosophy behind the training. Key players in the initial steering or support group may be able to reassure individuals or groups who perceive change as a threat to their power base. If action plans are developed within the training programme, the steering group may help staff to prioritize the ideas they have and to act on any further training and development needs that arise as a result of the initial training programme.

A management team, within the care setting, that is enthusiastic and committed to the training programme and developing the quality of their care will undoubtedly help to overcome and perhaps pre-empt obstacles. However, a management team that is divided or resistant to the ideas generated through training could create further problems. If an organization has a management team – for example, the owners of a small group of private homes or the middle management in social services or voluntary organizations – who are responsible for the care setting, committed to the training programme and in a position to help the care setting manager manage change then it may be possible to overcome obstacles created by resistant individuals or groups. If the manager is also the facilitator of the training, additional sources of support may be needed for the manager's message to be acted upon.

Resources are a key issue if staff have identified gaps in their own knowledge requiring further training and development input, or if their ideas to improve their care practice require an injection of funds. Organizations and homes work to a budget and the necessary financial resources may not be there. Staff at the care setting and organization levels may need to consult and prioritize ideas that require resources to operationalize. For example, if it has been suggested that a) a minibus is needed to take residents on outings and b) the garden requires work so as to encourage its use by residents, both of which require an injection of cash, then a decision must be reached as to which idea will be acted upon first.

Staff may need to think through alternative ways of obtaining the resources they need such as fund-raising. For fund-raising to be a success staff will need to be motivated and committed to their workplace. If support structures for staff are non-existent then it is likely that staff fund-raising initiatives will not receive the support of all staff. Yet there may be some members of staff who are committed, have spare time and are sufficiently inspired by the ideas they have helped to generate through training to spearhead a fund-raising campaign.

It can be seen that if the wider issues of recruitment and staff support systems are not addressed it will be difficult to overcome obstacles. Interim measures may address individual obstacles, and perhaps create new ones in the process, but a care setting which does not support its staff is likely to create long-term obstacles to change and the delivery of good-quality care. In such circumstances, an injection of training alone will not be sufficient.

SUGGESTED FURTHER READING

Although not about training, interested readers may find Halls (1997) discussion on organizations useful in illuminating problems they encounter in trying to promote change through training

Chapter 6

Evaluating the Training Programme

This chapter considers the final phase in the training process, evaluating the training programme. The training can be evaluated by all those involved in the process. The participants, the facilitator and perhaps the sponsor can all comment on its content and teaching style. The second way to evaluate the training is to assess the impact the training appears to have had on daily practice. The first type of evaluation is often carried out as a matter of routine. The second is an area that is relatively unexplored. Evaluating the impact training has had on practice can be achieved in a number of ways. First, the tactics of assessments and action plans built into the training programme can be examined to see if they have had an effect on practice; second, the care setting can be re-evaluated using techniques similar to those used in Phase 2, the 'getting to know the setting' phase of the training process. It is crucial that both of these components of training evaluation are incorporated if the aim of training is to equip the staff and organization to provide a high-quality service for the service users, people with dementia. I believe that organizations, large or small, have a responsibility not just to provide training to staff but to provide training that benefits the users of the service, people with dementia. If organizations can provide *evidence* that training is making a difference to care practice and the lives of people with dementia then training can be used as a strong marketing tool. The current climate surrounding service provision is to provide services that the user is satisfied with. Undoubtedly, training of staff is necessary to achieve this, but without an evaluation of the effects of training there is no evidence that this is the case.

EVALUATING THE TRAINING PROGRAMME

There are a number of people who can evaluate the training programme:

- the participants

- the facilitator

- an observer.

The most common way to evaluate training courses is for participants to complete a course evaluation form. Course evaluation forms vary in the questions they ask and the way in which questions are worded. Closed questions may encourage participants to complete the forms, as they tend to require less effort and thought to complete and are also easier to analyse. For example, if a yes/no answer format is utilized, a simple counting can take place. If four or five different responses are allowed a slightly more elaborate counting can occur, perhaps combining 'strongly agree' with 'agree' and 'strongly disagree' with 'disagree' and then calculating percentages to indicate what participants liked and did not like. Open-ended questions give participants a greater opportunity to say in their own words what they think about issues, but may take longer for participants to complete. Allocating time within a training session can overcome this. There remains, however, the issue of analysing the responses. Open-ended questions take much longer to analyse as each participant could, potentially, give a different answer, everyone of which needs careful grouping, coding and analysis.

The following boxes contain extracts from a closed course evaluation form containing leading questions, and questions of an open-ended format designed to encourage participants to comment on issues of their choice.

Course evaluation form

Please tick one box for each question

1. Overall, I enjoyed the course.   Yes ☐   No ☐

2. Overall, the teaching on the
course was of high quality.   Yes ☐   No ☐

3. I was interested in the content
of the course.   Yes ☐   No ☐

4. The course was well structured.   Yes ☐   No ☐

Figure 6.1 A closed course evaluation form

This form has numerous problems. Is it enough to know whether participants enjoyed the course? Is all learning enjoyable? Was the course designed to be enjoyable or to make people feel uncomfortable and 'move on' because of this? What does 'high quality' mean? Different individuals will interpret this in different ways, thus it is not a question that can be easily analysed. The third question gives no space for the participant to comment on the particular aspects of the content they may or may not have enjoyed. The final question again gives the participant no opportunity to reflect on the course as whole and state what they thought was well structured and what was not.

Course evaluation form

Course evaluation form

1. Did you attend the session on life-history? Yes/No

If yes, are there any comments you would like to make about content, teaching style or anything else?_____

_____

_____

_____

_____

2. Did you attend the session on care planning? Yes/No

If yes, are there any comments you would like to make about content, teaching style or anything else?_____

_____

_____

_____

_____

3. Did you attend the session on activities for people with dementia? Yes/No

If yes, are there any comments you would like to make about content, teaching style or anything else?_____

_____

_____

_____

_____

4. Are there any other comments you would like to make about the training? _____

_____

_____

_____

Figure 6.2 An open-ended course evaluation form

This second form is better than the first in a number of ways. It gives the participant an opportunity to say whether they attended specific sessions, and, if they wish, to comment upon them. In other words, participants are encouraged to say what they think. The final question gives the participant the opportunity to comment on anything about the training, so the venue and the length of breaks could be mentioned, as could the facilitator's teaching style, and perhaps any topics they would or would not recommend including in future courses.

An alternative and/or complementary way is for staff to discuss the course amongst themselves in the final part of a session and give verbal feedback to the facilitator, which is recorded (taped or scribed). Answers can be grouped together thematically to illustrate aspects of the course that staff were satisfied or dissatisfied with. These can be compared to the written responses of individuals. Participants may respond differently to the course depending on whether they can be identified, as in the case of verbal feedback, or remain anonymous, as is the case with written evaluation forms.

Evaluating the content, structure and modes of delivery as perceived by the participants on the course is important for all concerned in the training programme. Evaluation, verbal or written, provides the facilitator with feedback on what participants enjoyed, disliked or were indifferent to about the programme and, if necessary, can be used to help the facilitator change any aspect of the training. Those financing the training are also likely to be interested in the comments of participants. In addition, it is only fair to give participants the opportunity to comment on the training programme and for comments, positive, negative or indifferent, to be taken into account.

The facilitator should also evaluate the training programme. To achieve this it is helpful if the facilitator keeps a 'diary' record of each session. This should include information and reflections on who participated, the dynamics of the group, whether the time allocated to exercises was in line with the time participants required, which exercises appeared to engage participants, whether any issues required further clarification, and whether the trainer talked more than anyone else. The facilitator can use this self-reflective exercise to develop self-awareness and insight into the process of training. It also provides a useful comparison between participant and facilitator perspectives.

Another way of evaluating a programme which has been suggested is to have an 'independent observer' present throughout the course, who will provide feedback to the facilitator about the teaching materials, teaching style, and their impression of the group dynamics. There are problems with the notion of an observer who can be 'independent'. Anyone who observes a situation will form an impression which is partial and incomplete. The brief given to the 'independent observer' will have an effect on the type and quality of observations and the subsequent interpretations of what was observed. It may, however, be difficult to find any observer who can evaluate the programme fully, i.e. for content and for style. The evaluator may be in a position to comment on the materials, being aware of the issues covered, but may not understand teaching styles or learning styles. Alternatively, an evaluator may have knowledge of teaching and learning styles but have no knowledge of the content of the programme.

In addition to the immediate evaluation of the training by participants, it may be useful to evaluate the training six or twelve months after the event so as to monitor staff perceptions over time and ascertain whether the programme has had any effect on their practice and whether this has been long lasting. This would allow those involved in the earlier phase of 'getting started' to act if, for example, participants felt they needed a refresher course, or if a manager felt that the whole course should be delivered to new staff in the care setting. It would also give the initial steering/support group the opportunity to be proactive and plan future training in a way that takes account of the effects of time.

EVALUATING THE EFFECT OF ASSESSMENTS AND ACTION PLANS ON PRACTICE

The tactics discussed in chapter 5, of incorporating assessments into the training programme and helping staff to develop action plans, are designed to encourage participants to act upon the ideas discussed in training and can be evaluated at an agreed time period after the training has ended. A simple way to judge the effectiveness of assessments is to count the number of staff who have completed and passed the assessment. If staff did not meet the assessment criteria first time round it is good practice to offer them the opportunity to resubmit. If a number of staff do not manage to pass on their first attempt the facilitator may need to examine the assessment to ensure that the instructions are clear and that the information needed to complete the assessment is included in the training. It may be that staff invited to resubmit will choose not to do so; it is useful to explore the possible reasons for this decision with such members of staff and possibly the management team in the care setting. A member of staff who is having problems out of work may need support to complete the assessed work, perhaps through the allocation of a proportion of their work time to the assessment. In addition, it may be appropriate to examine whether the assessed work, in the example above a section of a care plan (see pp.68–70), is implemented into the regular care plan system of a home. It is also useful to explore the extent to which the plans staff developed for each person with dementia have actually been implemented. Staff may complete and pass the assessed work, but if it is not implemented into day-to-day practice then the exercise has not been truly effective.

Similarly, action plans are only useful if they are acted upon. The initial action plans developed during training are a starting point, but if they are to have an effect on practice the staff group will have to be committed and choose to discuss and develop their ideas further. Follow-up training sessions could be held to give staff the opportunity to discuss the progress of their action plans. The manager of a home may choose to set up meetings specifically to develop and monitor the action plans, or may incorporate the action plan as a regular item on the agenda of staff meetings. The facilitator or another member of the initial steering/support group for the training may use these opportunities to examine the impact action plans have had or are having on practice over time. At the outset of the training it may have been agreed that action plans would be reviewed perhaps three, six and twelve months after the training had ended. Reviewing the action plans could coincide with reviewing staff perceptions of the training and its relevance to their care practice. It is useful to explore the proportion of proposed actions that have been acted upon. This would give an indication of staff commitment and highlight areas requiring further support or resources if the proposed actions are to become a reality.

EVALUATING THE EFFECTS OF THE TRAINING PROGRAMME ON PRACTICE

The original methods used to get to know the setting in phase 2 of the training process can be employed to compare the setting as it was prior to and as it is after the training programme. It is helpful to have a small checklist of the key areas that it was hoped that the training would address. More formally, a list of potential or expected outcome measures may have been developed. There may, however, have been no preconceived ideas about outcomes, or differences in opinion as to what a 'successful' outcome may be. Any facilitator would be advised to include these issues in discussions held prior to the delivery of the training. This would later provide a starting point for a review of the setting as a whole and a detailed examination of the areas it was hoped that the training would directly influence.

Overtveit (1997) provides a comprehensive overview of ways to evaluate health interventions, which are readily transferable to the dementia care setting. There are, however, many pitfalls when evaluating any intervention or policy. One is that 'different people looking at the same data can come up with different conclusions' (Weiss 1972, p.32), for example, about how the training worked and what impact it has had. The way in which the evaluation is done will influence the eventual outcomes. This can be exemplified by using dementia-specific examples that build upon Ovreveit's (1997, pp.53–67) six types of evaluation:

1. descriptive

2. audit

3. before–after

4. comparative–experimentalist

5. randomized controlled trial or experiment

6. intervention to a health organization, including the impact on providers and the impact on users of the service receiving the intervention.

Descriptive and before–after type designs appear to be the most appropriate when evaluating a training programme, but each of Ovretveit's types of evaluation could be used. A *descriptive* evaluation would describe the content of the training and the facilitator's teaching style, and if Ovretveit's typology is followed then it may be similar to the example outlined above in which the training programme is evaluated from the point of view of all those who participated. This would give descriptive data about the training intervention incorporating individual participants' views.

The *before–after* design is appropriate if the facilitator has evaluated the setting at the 'getting to know the setting' phase and then evaluates the setting again after the training has taken place. For example, if Dementia Care Mapping is used as a tool to get to know the setting, the data for residents as a group prior to and after the training can be compared to see if there have been any changes in their well-being and in the main behaviours they engage in.

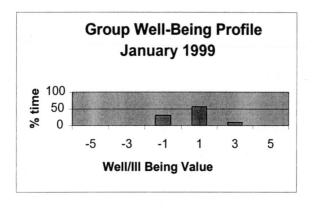

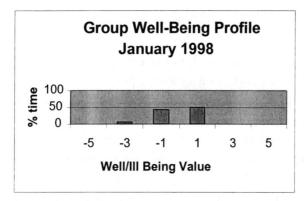

Figure 6.3 Comparison of group well-being profiles

Well-being values range from -5 to +5, the minus scores being an indication of ill-being and the positive scores of well-being. It can be seen that in 1999 residents as a group were in state of well-being for a larger amount of time.

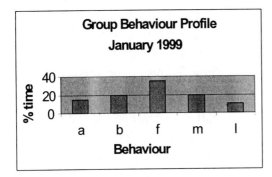

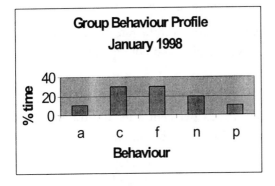

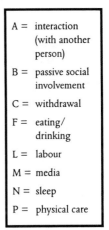

A = interaction (with another person)

B = passive social involvement

C = withdrawal

F = eating/ drinking

L = labour

M = media

N = sleep

P = physical care

Figure 6.4 Comparison of group behaviour profiles

It can be seen that the main categories of behaviour observed in 1998 and 1999 differ. In 1999 the active categories of labour and media are prominent. Residents are now socially alert rather than withdrawn and spend more time interacting with others.

The data in figures 6.3 and 6.4 would thus suggest that there has been an improvement in the well-being of people with dementia in the year that staff participated in a training programme. The training alone could not be held responsible for any changes, as life in residential and nursing homes constantly changes, and any other changes in the life of a home would need to be taken into account when interpreting the DCM data.

If an *audit*-type tool has been used, a comparison can be made not only with identified standards but with, for example, resident and staff turnover prior to and after the training, which may contribute to the presence or absence of any changes. Thus, in the year leading up to the training it may be found that staff turnover was high, 40 per cent, and in the year following the training had fallen to 15%. These figures can be interpreted in a number of ways:

1.   Prior to the training, staff were unsupported and had few training and development opportunities. The training may have encouraged staff to stay by creating the opportunity for staff to work together as a team and contribute to the planning of care.

2.   The training had no bearing on the rate of staff turnover. The first figures were a 'blip' and not representative of a typical year.

If staff turnover had been fairly low initially, for example at 10 per cent, and increased to 25 per cent after the training this could, again, be interpreted in a number of ways.

1.   The training encouraged staff to develop and move on to new things, perhaps further training and development.

2.   The training suggested a new way of working to which staff could not adhere.

Any findings are thus open to debate. When audit tools are used the whole picture needs to be examined. One piece of information, such as staff turnover, cannot be looked at in isolation from other variables. To expand on the second example above, in which an initial low staff turnover rate increased after the training, it may be that resident turnover increased markedly in the same time period. Staff who had been attached to the original client group may have been unwilling or unable to adjust to a new group of people with dementia and thus left the care setting. The reason for this would again be open to interpretation. It could be, for example, that staff were not given the support to work through their feelings of bereavement.

The third type of evaluation that Ovretveit describes, *comparative–experimentalist*, involves two different interventions being compared before and after their implementation. Thus two different training programmes would be introduced into two care settings and both compared prior to and after the intervention (the training programme). The same methods of evaluation would be used – perhaps an audit tool, Dementia Care Mapping, or both. It would be difficult to make conclusive comparisons based on any findings, as there may have been many other variables effecting the successes and failures observed. The training may not have been the only intervention or variable introduced into the care setting. A new manager can, for example, initiate many changes that may or may not be related to the training intervention.

In order to attempt to control variables other than the training itself, the evaluation may take the form of a *randomized control trial or experiment*. This involves randomly selecting two settings, often from a sample of similar care settings. One would receive the training and the other would not. Any changes observed in the setting receiving the training could then be attributed to the intervention. There are, however, problems with the approach, as again there may be other variables that change over time and, unlike a laboratory, care settings can be in a constant state of flux, the most obvious cause being when new staff, residents or relatives enter the home. Changes in shift patterns can have an effect, as can changes in meal times.

The sixth type of evaluation that Ovretveit suggests, *evaluating an intervention to a health organization*, has much currency at the moment. If the intervention can be shown to have had an impact on those receiving it and in turn to have had a beneficial effect upon the clients/users of the service then there may be commercial benefits. If training could be shown to benefit people with dementia then it could be surmised that the training is a 'good thing'. Benefits to people with dementia could be shown through DCM data, for example, as in the case of the before–after type evaluation outlined above.

Although Ovretveit distinguishes between types of evaluation it can be seen from the above that there are overlaps. The underlying philosophy of each type of evaluation is, however, of importance, as it will influence what interpretations can be drawn from the evaluation. In addition, the starting point of the person who initiates the evaluation will influence the type of evaluation they choose. People may choose the randomized control type of evaluation because of the high status the medical profession attributes to randomized control trials. Alternatively, someone may choose an audit evaluation if they believe they have a set of existing high standards and wish to compare them with those of another setting at one point in time and/or over time.

Thus, deciding on a technique with which to evaluate the impact of training on care practice is not easy. This does not mean that evaluation should not be attempted, only that whoever uses evaluation information must be aware that many inferences can be drawn depending on how the data are interpreted. In addition, it must be remembered that those who are evaluated will 'destroy the credibility of the message' if they feel they have something to lose from the evaluation (Ovretveit 1997, p.188). This can occur regardless of the type of evaluation used. Therefore, any changes or constants over the evaluation period are open to individuals' interpretations, as are explanations of why changes did or did not occur. Just as statements of policy may be a means of demonstrating that something is being done to ease the situation (Parsons 1995, p.612) buying in or providing in-house training may be a means of demonstrating a commitment to change even when none is desired or regarded as possible.

In a more positive vein, it is hoped that the purpose of the evaluation will be to improve service provision for people with dementia and to equip staff to do this. Therefore, those who refer to evaluation information will often use it to plan and improve the service they provide. Evaluation is only of value when those who look at the information judge it to be so.

Evaluation may be the end point for some people, but if the whole process of training is to be effective then the evaluation phase requires one further consideration: based on the information the evaluation has generated, what should be done next?

SUMMING UP

'What should be done next?' is a crucial question to ask during the final phase of the training process. The successful delivery of the training programme (Phase 4) and positive evaluation (Phase 6) of the course may suggest that the training programme is a useful product. Participants may begin to implement ideas discussed within training through assessed pieces of work, personal pledges and, perhaps, group action plans (Phases 5 and 6). However, the training process as a whole can be undermined if staff do not receive support and are not encouraged to act on the training. The sixth phase may identify areas requiring attention, and if further plans are not developed to maintain the momentum then the successes of the previous phases will not be sustained.

It may be decided that a one-off training session should be arranged to give staff the opportunity to raise any outstanding issues or concerns. This is a short-term measure that may be required but which does not ensure the ongoing development of care practice. A series of follow-up training sessions is another option that is fairly easy to operationalize. For these to be relevant to the current climate in a setting and the needs of staff and residents at a particular point in time then some kind of synthesis of the above phases may be required at regular intervals. For example, another Dementia Care Mapping evaluation may be carried out to ascertain the current well-being of a number of people with dementia within a setting just before a follow-up training session.

If staff have developed an action plan, the home and/or organization may have to explore resource implications and decide whether the ideas staff suggested are priorities and then how to act on them. In addition, issues may have emerged which apply to the organization as a whole.

The original facilitator may or may not be involved in subsequent discussions arising from the initial training, and a different facilitator may be brought in to work with staff on issues brought up during the evaluation phase of the process. The training phase outlined in this guide is therefore a *cyclical* process. The final aspect of Phase 6 is, essentially, concerned with taking stock of where the training has taken the care setting and then identifying further action required for

- individual staff development needs

- the development needs of the staff group

- the development needs of the care setting

- and, perhaps the development needs of the organization as a whole.

Thus, training is not, as may initially be thought by some, a simple exercise of parachuting into and then running out of a care setting with the hope that information delivered will be taken on-board and used. This guide has illustrated the complexities that facilitators of training may find they have to deal with. The process of training begins not at the delivery phase or even the design phase, but when an initial suggestion is made that training may be necessary. Delivering effective training and evaluating whether or not training has been effective are not simple matters. Many aspects require consideration. The design and delivery of the training programme are of course crucial parts of the process, but without prior knowledge of issues such as the culture of the care setting, the politics of the organization, and the reason(s) for deciding to give staff training it will be difficult to judge what is needed (Phases 1 and 2). If measures are not built into the design of the training programme that encourage the incorporation into care practice and development of ideas discussed in training, can the training be judged to be effective? The issue of evaluation is a crucial element of training programmes of any kind. In the continually developing field of dementia care there is a need to find out what works for people with dementia. At this point in time there is much uncertainty as to what constitutes high-quality care and whether current standards are in line with the needs of the users and providers of the service. Training in itself will not resolve these wider issues, but the process of training can be used to inform the debate.

References

Aronson, M.K. (1994) *Reshaping Dementia Care: Practice and Policy in Long Term Care.* California: Sage.

Benner, P. (1984) *From Novice to Expert: Excellence and Power in Clinical Nursing Practice.* Menlo Park, USA: Addison Wesley Publishing Company.

Bowie, P. and Mountain, G. (1993) 'Using direct observation methods to record the behaviour of long stay patients with dementia.' *International Journal of Geriatric Psychiatry 8,* 857–864.

Bradford Dementia Group (1997) *Evaluating Dementia Care: The DCM Method.* Bradford: University of Bradford.

Bramley, P. (1991) *Evaluating Training Effectiveness: Translating Theory into Practice.* London: McGraw-Hill.

Brooker, D.J.R. (1995) 'Looking at them, looking at me: A review of observational studies into the quality of institutional care for elderly people with dementia.' *Journal of Mental Health 4,* 145–156.

Brooker, D.J.R., Foster, N., Banner, A., Payne, M. and Jackson, L. (1998) 'The efficacy of dementia care mapping as an audit toll: Report of a three year British NHS evaluation.' *Ageing and Mental Health, 2,* 1, 60–70.

Burnard, P. (1989) *Teaching Interpersonal Skills: A Handbook of Experiential Learning for Health Professionals.* London: Chapman and Hall.

Cohen-Mansfield, J. (1989) 'Sources of satisfaction and stress in nursing home care-givers: Preliminary results.' *Journal of Advanced Nursing 14,* 383–388.

Cross, P. (1981) *Adults as Learners.* San Fransisco: Jossey Bass.

Dawson, S. (1996) *Analysing Organisations.* Basingstoke: Macmillan.

Dean, R., Proudfoot, R. and Lindesay, J. (1993) 'The quality of interactions schedule (QUIS): development, reliability and use in the evaluation of two domus units.' *International Journal of Geriatric Psychiatry 8,* 819–826.

Derbyshire, P. (1994) 'Skilled expert practice: is it all in the mind? A response to English's critique of Benner's novice to expert model.' *Journal of Advanced Nursing 19,* 755–761.

English, J. (1993) 'Intuition as a function of the expert nurse: a critique of Benner's novice to expert model.' *Journal of Advanced Nursing 18*, 387–393.

Frazier, C. and Sherlock, L. (1994) 'Staffing patterns and training for competent dementia care.' In M. K. Aronson (ed.) *Reshaping Dementia Care: Practice and Policy in Long Term Care.* California: Sage.

Gerrish, K., McManus, M. and Ashworth, P. (1997) *Researching Professional Education: Levels of Achievement: A Review of the Assessment of Practice.* London: English National Board for Nursing, Midwifery and Health Visiting.

Goffman, E. (1961) *Asylums.* Harmondsworth: Pelican.

Goldsmith, M. (1996) *Hearing the Voice of People with Dementia.* London: Jessica Kingsley Publishers.

Hall, R.H. (1997) *Organizations: Structures, Processes and Outcomes.* London: Prentice Hall.

Hammersley, M. and Atkinson, P. (1983) *Ethnography: Principles in Practice.* London: Tavistock.

Handy, C. (1993) *Understanding Organizations.* Harmondsworth: Penguin.

Hockey, J. (1990) *Experiences of Death.* Edinburgh: Edinburgh University Press.

Honey, P. and Mumford, A. (1982) *The Manual of Learning Styles.* Maidenhead.

Hopkins, A., Brocklehurst, J. and Dickinson, E. (1992) *The CARE Scheme: Continuous Assessment Review and Evaluation.* London: Royal College of Physicians.

Hyland, T. (1993) 'Professional development and competence-based education.' *Educational Studies 19*, 1, 123–132.

Illich, I. (1971) *Celebration of Awareness.* Harmondsworth: Penguin.

Innes, A. (1998) *A Structural Audit Tool for Dementia Care Settings.* University of Bradford: Bradford.

Jasper, M. A. (1994) 'Expert: A discussion of the implications of the concept as used in nursing.' *Journal of Advanced Nursing 20*, 769–776.

Killick, J. (1997), *You are Words.* London: Hawker Publications.

Kitwood, T. (1995) 'Cultures of care: Tradition and change.' In T. Kitwood and S. Benson (eds) *The New Culture of Dementia Care.* London: Hawker Publications.

Kitwood, T. (1998) 'Professional and moral development for care work: Some observations of the process.' *The Journal of Moral Education 27*, 3, 401–411.

Kitwood, T. and Bredin, K. (1992a) *Person to Person: A Guide to the Care of those with Failing Mental Powers*. Essex: Gale Publications.

Kitwood, T. and Bredin, K. (1992b) *Evaluating Dementia Care: The DCM Method*. University of Bradford: Bradford Dementia Group.

Kitwood, T. and Woods, B. (1996) *Training and Development Strategy for Dementia Care in Residential Settings*. University of Bradford: Bradford Dementia Group.

Knowles, M. (1970) *The Modern Practice of Adult Education*. New York: Association Press.

Kolb, D.A. (1984) *Experiential Learning: Experience as the Source of Learning and Development*. New York: Prentice Hall.

Lee-Treweek, G. (1997) 'Emotion work, order and emotional power in care assistant work.' In N James (ed.) *The Sociology of Health and the Emotions*. Oxford: Blackwell.

Loveday, B., Kitwood, T. and Bowe, B. (1998) *Improving Dementia Care*. London: Hawker Publications.

May, T. (1993) *Social Research*. Buckingham: Open University Press.

MacDonald, A.J.D., Craig, T.K.L. and Warner, L.A.R. (1985) 'The development of a short observation method for the study of activity and contacts of old people in residential settings.' *Psychological Medicine 15*, 167–172.

McCrane, E.W., Lambert, V.A. and Lambert, C.E. (1987) 'Work stress, hardiness and burnout among hospital staff nurses.' *Nursing Research 36* 6, 374–378.

Moniz-Cooke, E.D., Agar, S., Silver, M., Woods, R., Wang, M., Elston, C. and Win, T, (1998) 'Can staff training reduce carer stress and behavioural disturbance in the elderly mentally ill?' *International Journal of Geriatric Psychiatry 13*, 149–158.

Moos, R.H. and Lemke, S. (1992) *Multiphasic Environmental Assessment Procedure (MEAP) Users Guide*. California: Centre for Health Care Evaluation.

Murphy, C. (1994) *It Started With a Sea Shell*. University of Stirling: Dementia Services Development Centre.

Oppenheim, A.N. (1966) *Questionnaire Design and Attitude Measurement*. London: Heinemann.

Ovretveit, J. (1997) *Evaluating Health Interventions*. Buckingham: Open University Press.

Parsons, W. (1995) *Public Policy*. Aldershot: Edward Elgar.

Power, M. (1997) *The Audit Society*. Oxford: Oxford University Press.

Rogers, A. (1986) *Teaching Adults*. Buckingham: Open University Press.

Schon, D.A. (1983) *The Reflective Practitioner*. London: Arena.

Schon, D.A. (1987) *Educating the Reflective Practitioner.* San Francisco: Jossey Bass.

Weiner, R. (1997) *Creative Training: Sociodrama and Team-building.* London: Jessica Kingsley Publishers.

Weiss, C.H. (1972) *Evaluation Research: Methods of Assessing Program Effectiveness.* Englewood Cliffs, NJ: Prentice Hall.

Willcocks, D., Peace, S. and Kellaher, L. (1987) *Private Lives in Public Places.* London: Tavistock.

Wilkinson, A.M. (1993) 'Dementia care mapping: A pilot study of its implementation in a psychogeriatric service.' *International Journal of Geriatric Psychiatry 8,* 1027–1029.

Subject Index

Author Index